SIX-FOOT TIGER, THREE-FOOT CAGE

TAKE CHARGE OF YOUR HEALTH BY
TAKING CHARGE OF YOUR MOUTH

*Holistic Mouth Solutions for
Sleep Apnea, Deficient Jaws, and
Related Complications*

DR. FELIX LIAO, DDS

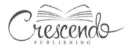

Crescendo
PUBLISHING

Six-Foot Tiger, Three-Foot Cage:
Take Charge of Your Health by Taking Charge of Your Mouth
by Dr. Felix Liao

Cover Design By Melody Hunter

ISBN: 978-1-944177-59-1 (p)
ISBN: 978-1-944177-60-7 (e)
ISBN: 978-1-944177-83-6 (P-Color)

Crescendo Publishing, LLC
300 Carlsbad Village Drive
Ste. 108A, #443
Carlsbad, California 92008-2999
1-877-575-8814

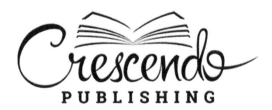

PUBLISHING

A Note from the Author

The mouth structure is a hugely important but much overlooked part of total health and natural wellness. Snoring, teeth grinding, chronic fatigue, persistent pains, sleep apnea, and their related complications can be rooted in an impaired mouth handicapping whole body health.

"Three-foot cage" in this book's title represents underdeveloped jaws. "Six-foot tiger" refers to the vicious physical and financial consequences of an impaired mouth. You can take off your high heels or pinchy glasses when you get home, but you can't remove an impaired mouth when you go to sleep -- until now.

A Holistic Mouth has the right ingredients and structural form to support the airway for oxygen delivery and nourishing sleep. It thus provides a consistently effective and natural solution to a surprising range of health troubles. Impaired Mouth Syndrome is not yet a formal diagnosis, but my term for describing the diverse medical, dental, and mood symptoms associated with an impaired mouth that can eat, drink, talk, but cannot support airway, sleep, and structural alignment.

I write this book to help you connect the dots with scientific evidence and common sense, and to see how overall health can improve when an impaired mouth is treated with Holistic Mouth Solutions in real-life cases. No part of this book is intended as medical or dental advice. Please consult your own health professional(s) regarding your symptoms and questions.

I recommend that you read the chapters in the order presented, starting with the Introduction, for best results. Additional information and resources for consumers and healthcare professionals are available at www.HolisticMouthSolutions.com.

An impaired mouth is a slow kill, whereas a Holistic Mouth is a fast heal. I hope this new awareness will lead to better health and higher life quality for many people with help from you, my readers.

Praise for Six-Foot Tiger, Three-Foot Cage

"In *Six-Foot Tiger, Three-Foot Cage,* Dr. Felix Liao demonstrates conclusively the vital yet little understood link between the structure and form of the oral cavity and general health. Understanding and properly addressing this connection can solve many problems that most physicians today still consider difficult or even impossible to effectively treat.

Dr. Liao is a gifted educator, and he has a clear and very readable style of writing. His work effectively expands on many of the concepts promoted years ago by the brilliant Dr. Weston Price. Combined with the increasingly recognized cause-and-effect relationship between occult dental infections and chronic disease, it becomes clear that optimizing the health and structure of the mouth and oral cavity is of paramount importance in effectively treating any chronically ill patient. Kudos to Dr. Liao for this wonderful book."

Thomas E. Levy, MD, JD
Author of *Uninformed Consent, Death by Calcium*

"The very clear text and illustrations in *Six-Foot Tiger, Three-Foot Cage* make it an excellent read for patients and professionals. Thank you Dr. Liao for teaching both children and adults the significant harm that skeletal malocclusions exert on the body, and helping them not only find their orthopedically-correct bite with oral expansion appliances, but also at the deepest level - their true self."

Louisa L. Williams, MS, DC, ND
Author of *Radical Medicine*

"I highly recommend this revolutionary book by Dr. Liao because it's time to put an end to the suffering by patients and their families stemming from craniofacial deficiencies. *Six-Foot Tiger, Three-Foot Cage* connects the dots between underlying etiology and clinical signs and symptoms, and offers both solutions and life stories that illustrate the importance of oral health that supports whole body health."

G. Dave Singh, DDSc, PhD, DMD
Author of *Epigenetic Orthodontics in Adults*

"As a surgeon who specializes in sex hormone endocrinology effecting health and aging, it became evident in our clinic that the most common relationship of **low testosterone in young men was sleep apnea.**

Correcting body structural abnormalities, adjusting hormonal imbalances and insulin metabolism, nasal airway obstructions and oral pharyngeal airway obstructions are more fundamental than to just prescribe CPAP airway aids.

Dr. Felix Liao, a disciple of the legendary Dr. Weston Price, is a dentist with a special focus on oral airway obstructions and has the artful skills to reshape the Maxilla and Mandible jaw structures to accommodate the tongue positions leading to airway obstructions - *thus the release of the "Six-Foot Tiger" tongue trapped in a "Three-Foot Cage" mouth and jaw.*

Without major surgery, his artful skill to use expandable oral appliances to correct malfunctions is an important contribution to medicine.

The book is readable for laymen, dentists and other professionals and makes us all aware of how important oral airways can effect major metabolic and physical abnormalities and finally to disease states. The clarity and simplicity of his arguments are supported by the large body of references for professional corroboration.

We should all read this book!

George Yu,
Clinical Professor of Urological Surgery, George Washington
University Medical Center, Sex hormone Endocrinology, Aegis
Medical & Research Associates,
Yufoundation.org

"The doctors who read and internalize the concepts in *Six-Foot Tiger, Three-Foot Cage* will increase their diagnostic abilities and treatment results at least 50 fold. This book should be mandatory reading for all medical and dental professionals. I wish I had written it myself at the beginning of my career."

Brendan C. Stack, DDS, MS,
Orthodontist and TMJ Specialist

"It's time to sit up and pay attention to Dr. Liao's point: an Impaired Mouth is the start of a domino leading to medical, dental, mental, and financial troubles. I strongly recommend you find out why and how by reading *Six-Foot Tiger, Three-Foot Cage*."

Sally Fallon Morell, President
The Weston A. Price Foundation

"Doctor Liao's new book, *Six-Foot Tiger, Three-Foot Cage* was so engaging, I read it in one sitting. Indeed, AIRWAY rules sleep, which in turn drives energy, healing and total health.

Doctor Liao's innovative thoughts reflect a paradigm shift in Dentistry from tooth health to "WholeHealth". So, we tell our orthodontic students, that medical and dental care should start with an assessment of airway and sleep as well as mouth structure.

Whether you are health provider or layperson, if you care about health and life quality, the forward thinking ideas presented will be well worth the read."

Richard T. Beistle, D.D.S.,
Developer of the Sassouni-Plus cephalometric analysis,
Instructor in orthodontic diagnosis for United States Dental
Institute and Straight Wire Orthodontic Studies.

"As a holistic MD, I often wonder why certain people don't get well despite good diet, supplements, detoxing and attention to their mental/emotional and spiritual health. Dr. Felix Liao's book *Six-Foot Tiger, Three-Foot Cage* brilliantly explains why. By weaving amazing case studies and compelling research, Dr. Liao has written a ground-breaking book that everyone, especially physicians and dentists, should read. I truly believe that this could be the missing piece of the puzzle for sufferers of chronic pain, chronic fatigue, sleep apnea/snoring and much more."

Margaret Gennaro, MD

"Great book! Dr. Liao's Six-Foot Tiger, Three-Foot Cage brilliantly connects snoring, sleep apnea, teeth grinding, chronic pain and fatigue with deficient mouth structure. It also convincingly shows Holistic Mouth is a natural solution for many medical and dental symptoms while you sleep - what a novel and yet sensible idea?! Holistic Mouth is indeed foundational to natural health and this book is a must read for everyone interested in natural health and wellness. This book helps me look deeper in to correlation between dental issues and overall health of my patients."

Dr. Sheri Salartash,
Family Dentist, Alexandria, VA

"I see myself in several of the cases in this book and am so grateful that my physician referred me to Dr. Liao. Even though I was in my late sixties, Dr. Liao's identification and treatment of several problems has me sleeping, breathing and walking better as I enter my 70's. So glad this book will help others identify possible causes of chronic conditions.

During my first consultation, Dr. Liao connected these dots for me: mouth-airway-sleep, and bite-spine-gait. At that time, I basically limped to favor my hurting and weak left knee, which had not responded to physical therapy after arthroscopic surgery.

My borderline sleep apnea was successfully treated by Dr. Liao's Holistic Mouth Solutions that widened my narrow palate so I can breathe through my nose and keep my mouth closed 24/7. In less than a year, I was breathing better, sleeping better, and finally dreaming again!

Redeveloping my narrow jaws and realigning my bite also improved my mobility. Dr. Liao referred me to a WholeHealth acupuncturist and the combination makes me feel and walk like I am years younger. Thank you Dr. Liao for helping to put the spring back in my step!"

S.C.,
Retired librarian

"6T3C by Dr. Felix Liao, DDS is one of the most comprehensive book written on mouthful evidence of connection between oral cavity, dental distress and unrecognized medical conditions. One of the hardest part of the medical evaluation and treatment plan is recognizing the hidden dental problems, and the reasons why patients are not responding to the standard medical care. Dr. Felix Liao explains clearly and in-depth why and how to fix the underlying dental related incurable medical conditions. This book is a must read for all dentists and medical doctors, and also, for patients with incurable medical conditions."

Simon Yu, MD,
Board Certified Internal Medicine,
Author of *Accidental Cure*

Dr. Liao is that rare dentist that truly understands the how the mouth inter-relates with the entire body. His *Six-Foot Tiger, Three-Foot Cage* brilliantly connects snoring, sleep apnea, teeth grinding, chronic pain and fatigue with having a mouth too small for the tongue. His unique insights ingeniously pull together tomes of published research along with years of clinical experience into his novel and sensible Holistic Mouth solution. A must read for anyone who wants to keep breathing naturally.

Steven Y. Park, MD.
Author of, *Sleep Interrupted:*
A physician reveals the #1 reason why so many of us are sick and
tired.

I have gotten to know Dr. Felix Liao very well as he has attended virtually all of my Ortho and TMD courses over the last eight years. I have great respect for his intensity and dedication to learning and to his desire to share his knowledge with others. Felix is one of the pioneers of the Holistic approach and I heartily recommend his new book, *Six Foot Tiger, Three Foot Cage*.

Dr. Jay W. Gerber,
Director of Instruction, Straight Wire Orthodontic Studies

As Dr. Liao's patient, I have personally experienced the positive results described in 6T3C, including deeper sleep, dreaming more, and having more energy for my workouts. This book is a must-read for all who suffer from undiagnosed Impaired Mouth Syndrome and their dentists and health professionals.

Hilda Labrada Gore,
Body & Soul Regional Director, Integrative Nutrition Health
Coach,
Wise Traditions Podcast Host

Disclaimer

The opinions, advice and recommendations in this book are intended for a wide audience of people and are not tailored or specific to any individual needs or health conditions.

This book is not intended as a substitute for professional medical or dental advice, diagnosis, or treatment. Always seek professional medical advice from your dentist, physician or other qualified heath care provider with any questions you may have regarding a medical condition. This book is not intended to diagnose, treat or cure any disease. Significant changes in your health regime should be discussed with your health care provider.

The authors and publishers of this book make no warranty, representation, or guarantee regarding the advice given in this book, nor do they assume any liability whatsoever arising out of your use of any information or product referenced in this book.

Any reproduction, retransmission, or republication (in whole or in part) of any document or information found in this book is expressly prohibited, unless we grant you consent in writing.

Table of Contents

Introduction

How Your Mouth
Drives Your Health

The mouth is the center of communication and contact. Along with the eyes, ears, and nose, it is positioned near the brain, ensuring close integration and coordination. We use the craniofacial complex— the oral, dental, and the other craniofacial tissues that house the organs of taste, vision, hearing, and smell—to experience and interact with the world around us.

– Oral Health in America:
A Report of the Surgeon General [1]

Your mouth is the gateway to your body and a critical infrastructure that supports sleep and supplies oxygen to your heart, brain, and teeth. That makes your mouth a crucial starting place for turning back illness and turning on wellness—that's the point of this book.

You are about to discover how to take fuller charge of your health by way of your mouth. For instance:

- Do you suffer from snoring, sleep apnea, teeth grinding, chronic pain, fatigue, moodiness, or one dental problem after another?

- Do you live with or know someone who does?

- Would like your children to grow without these troubles?

All mouths are not created equal. Is your mouth a health asset or a liability? If you're like most Americans, your mouth is likely not structurally fit to fulfill all its job descriptions on behalf of your health.

Simply put, a Holistic Mouth promotes overall health, while an impaired mouth is a handicap. It is important to know this because your mouth is a master driver of either your health or your health problems.

Going Wholistic

Your mouth has a far greater impact on your health than you and your health professionals realize. Holistic Mouth Solutions™ is a book series and a website connecting your mouth with your overall health like never before. Book 1 will look at your mouth's role in airway obstruction and quality sleep. We will connect the dots between impaired oral structure, airway obstruction, and the resulting medical, dental, and mood symptoms. You will see credible scientific evidence and unexpected improvements in oral-systemic health through real-life cases.

The title of this book, Six-Foot Tiger, Three-Foot Cage, is a metaphor for the many unrecognized cases of living with a normal "size 6" tongue in an underdeveloped "size 3" space framed by two deficient jaws. When the tongue's habitat is too small, it is forced into the throat where it clogs the airway and becomes a "tiger" that threatens life and stresses the body, fogs the mind, and grinds the teeth.

This airway obstruction by the tongue causes cumulative oxygen deficiency day and night, as well as poor sleep year after year, until it leads to various symptoms throughout the body. You will learn what those symptoms are and discover the surprisingly broad range of whole-body benefits that Holistic Mouth Solutions can provide.

In addition, you have just stepped into the WholeHealth movement in health care that is enabling people to reclaim their natural health far more efficiently than ever. WholeHealth is a "wholistic" view that sees all parts of the body as interconnected and mutually supportive — without departmental lines, super egos, and special interests. In WholeHealth, symptoms are properly seen as reactions, and removing an impaired mouth as a health blocker can resolve many symptoms, minimize recurrence, and downstream costs.

Recognition: The Mouth as a Health-Problem Source

The body wants peace when it sleeps, not a tiger tongue blocking the throat. Deep sleep can heal almost anything, provided the airway is open to deliver oxygen on demand, which in turn cannot afford a six-foot tiger in a three-foot cage.

Few health professionals are aware that an impaired mouth structure (deep overbite, weak chin, sunken midface, narrow jaws, crowded teeth, double chin, tongue-tie, and so on) can be the source of many medical, dental, mood, and life-quality problems, and even fewer know how to solve them at the source. But that's not their fault.

Odds are that the mouth was missing in their training and thus is missing in their thinking. Nonetheless, science is evolving and expanding the boundaries of the "old box." This book introduces Holistic Mouth Solutions as an efficient answer to many symptoms that defy resolution by traditional care.

Holistic Mouth is a brand-new concept and a new solution made possible by the advent of digital imaging, sleep medicine, epigenetics, craniofacial orthopedics, and the integration of many health professionals' expertise.

If you just can't get well, despite trying various symptom-management attempts, *Six-Foot Tiger, Three-Foot Cage* may be just what your health has been waiting for. It shows you how to start your health makeover with a wider airway for better sleep. You will see what happens to your overall health when that three-foot cage is redeveloped, resulting in a widened airway and huge upgrades in sleep quality. I will take you through my CSIs (chair-side investigations) that combine published evidence with case studies to illustrate crucial—and yet little-noticed—mind-body-mouth connections.

As a holistic dentist, I have a particular interest in the mouth's many roles in our overall health. "Holistic" is rooted in the ancient Greek concept of holism, or the whole made of mind, body, and spirit. Holistic Mouth™ is a term I coined to call attention to the mouth's pivotal role in our overall health.

Briefly, a Holistic Mouth has the necessary structural form to support basic health functions, including your ABCDES: alignment, breathing, circulation, digestion, energy, and sleep.

By contrast, an impaired mouth can eat, drink, talk, and even smile, but its deficient structure blocks ABCDES because it comes with a narrow airway, poor sleep, and premature degeneration from oxygen deficiency.

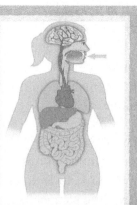

A Holistic Mouth Promotes Total Health and Life Quality

in terms of

- Alignment w/o pain in head, jaws, body
- Breathing w/o airway obstruction
- Circulation w/o dental infections
- Digestion w/o harmful toxins
- Energy w/o stimulants or chocolates
- Sleep w/o snoring, apnea, or teeth grinding

Green: breathing; Yellow: digestion; Red: circulation

As a family dentist, I help make teeth and gums healthy so that they can serve as a foundation of the Holistic Mouth.

As a Holistic Mouth doctor, I help to develop the mouth structures orthopedically and functionally to better support overall health. I connect the mouth with patients' medical, dental, and mood complaints and identify how each patient's diet, lifestyle, posture, habits, and overall health affect their sleep, airway, dental, and gum problems, and vice versa. I also refer patients to integrative health professionals as needed for the expertise beyond my scope of practice.

Better Sleep with Holistic Mouth? Definitely!

Holistic Mouth is a simple concept and a powerful solution. Better health comes naturally when the mouth has the right form (structures) to support ABCDES. Redeveloping deficient jaws with crowded teeth can liberate your tiger tongue, keeping it out of your airway so that you can sleep better.

An impaired mouth comes with a pinched airway from an underdeveloped cranio-dental-facial skeleton. "Development" here refers to a change in size and shape of a structure over time, such as a broader upper jaw (maxilla), lower jaw (mandible), and a wider airway inside the nose, behind the palate and the tongue, or all the above.

The good news? Impaired mouth structure in adults can now be redeveloped to mitigate snoring, sleep apnea, teeth grinding, aches and pains, and related medical and dental problems. This is done by signaling stem cells in and around the jaws and inside tooth sockets.

The mouth structure is a much bigger player in our total health and natural wellness than most patients and health professionals realize. Through these pages, you will learn:

1. How the medical, dental, and mental symptoms that appear to be difficult to treat can be caused by an impaired mouth structure that has gone undiagnosed

2. How to recognize an impaired mouth as the owner of your own body

3. What can be done to restore Holistic Mouth and how seemingly unrelated symptoms go away naturally.

Unlike any book before it, *Six-Foot Tiger, Three-Foot Cage* shows you—and your health professionals—precisely how to succeed at accomplishing a natural health upgrade by Holistic Mouth. This book is my answer to these frequent questions many health-conscious people like you have: "Why do I still suffer fatigue, aches and pains, depression, anxiety, high blood pressure, etc. despite faithful diet and exercise, yoga, meditation, supplements, flossing, and oil pulling?" or simply "Why don't I ever feel better?! I know something is not right, but my medical and dental checkups don't find anything wrong."

Recognizing and treating an impaired mouth structure that you never knew you had may very well be the start of a natural solution to those problems.

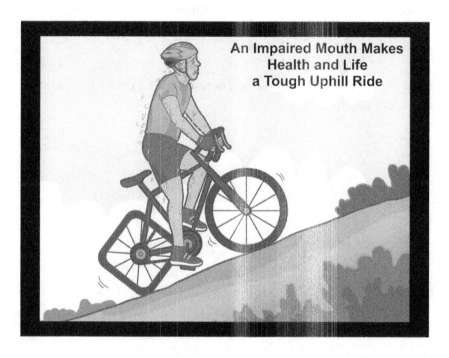

In summary, a Holistic Mouth is a health builder while an impaired mouth is a troublemaker. With a Holistic Mouth, whole-body health has a strong chance. With an impaired mouth, top-quality health remains out of reach.

Holistic Mouth: An Effective Solution

Turning an impaired mouth into a Holistic Mouth can be an effective solution for many symptoms in and around the mouth and often throughout the body. Consider Luke who, at age nine, had an overbite, a facial tic from Tourette syndrome, buck teeth, chronic mouth breathing, and low energy. All of this was interfering with his health and schooling. A year after starting treatment though, Luke was 100 percent free of his facial tic. Two and a half years later, he became a straight-A student taking advanced math and language-arts courses and playing tennis.

"I drove four hours each way [every other month] over these years," says Luke's dad on camera, "and I'm really proud that he's doing so well."

Luke says, "I feel I have lots of energy, and it's easier to learn now, and I feel happier."

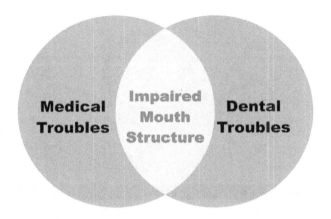

When the tongue's habitat is too small, it is forced into the throat, blocking the airway and causing stress from oxygen deficiency day and night. What if Luke were to graduate, go to work, and start a family without ever having his impaired mouth treated? Imagine the harmful effects it would have on his quality of life—not to mention his health-care costs!

Early recognition and treatment of an impaired mouth makes it possible to accomplish more with less effort, add years to your life, and bring life to your years.

And if your development years are behind you? Today, this is no longer a problem. Stem cells inside and around your jaws can be "switched on" to redevelop that size 3 cage to suit a size 6 tongue, which can spur a cascade of positive changes: the airway widens, sleep works, energy recovers, performance shines, facial radiance appears naturally, and, in turn, your overall health and well-being improve.

Holistic Mouth is a natural solution that can effectively release the body from the tyranny of persistent pain and the ravages of oxygen deficiency—without side effects—regardless of age, as long as you have enough good teeth in the right places. This is the WholeHealth difference, and a recurring theme in this book.

Better yet, achieving Holistic Mouth is a new, natural solution that takes place while you sleep. Best of all, Holistic Mouth requires no medication, surgery, drilling, or injections in uncomplicated cases.

Filling Knowledge Gaps Instead of Cavities

You can have physical, mental-emotional, or dental problems, but they are usually treated separately even though they share the same physical address. I write *Six-Foot Tiger, Three-Foot Cage* to:

- Fill a huge awareness gap: An impaired mouth is a barrier to total health and a frequently overlooked source of medical, dental, and mental health troubles

- Focus attention on the mouth's pivotal role in our overall health and natural wellness based on evidence and experience

- Help readers see the WholeHealth logic and whole-body benefits of connecting their medical and dental symptoms with their sleep, airway, and mouth structure

- Stimulate further research and training programs to help more patients achieve whole- health through Holistic Mouth, and vice versa

Join me on a surprising journey toward a huge improvement in your health by mouth, in the health of those you love, and if you are a health-care professional, in the health of your patients.

Holistic Mouth Bites

At the end of each chapter, I offer a few Holistic Mouth Bites— "take-away pearls" from the WholeHealth perspective, which sees the body not as a collection of parts for specialists to fix but as an integration of interconnected parts and systems.

Holistic Mouth Bites do not constitute medical or dental advice. They are simply conclusions that have made sense to me and worked for my patients. Although they have not been validated by formal studies, beware of opinions to the contrary offered by those with less or no clinical experience.

Until all the studies are in, one useful yardstick is your common sense. Asking yourself, "Does this make common sense?" is a good start.

Chapter One

Redeveloping an Impaired Mouth Benefits the Whole Body: The Case of Smithy

Different outcome requires different thinking.

— Thomas M. Rau, MD,
Medical Director, Paracelsus Klinik, Switzerland

Smithy, age thirty-six, came in initially for a toothache. Then she told me about her other symptoms that had been bothering her every day for years: pain in her mouth and gums, random gurgling sounds in her stomach, constant tiredness, and neck, shoulder, and wrist pain.

I suspected an impaired mouth and airway obstruction. Her Epworth Sleepiness Score (an accepted self-survey for sleep apnea) was 14—well above the threshold of 10, which suggests sleep apnea.[1] Her

CT scan showed her airway was in the red zone—the danger zone—and thus susceptible to collapse during sleep.

After a detailed consultation, Smithy elected to start treatment using oral appliances to redevelop her jaws, bite, and airway to help her sleep better. Her instructions included wearing her appliances fourteen to sixteen hours a day, including when she slept but excluding office hours.

Four months later, Smithy reported a 50 percent drop in her neck, shoulder, and carpal-tunnel pain, a 60 percent drop in her stress-related mouth pain, a 70 percent drop in her stomach symptoms, and an 80 percent drop in fatigue.

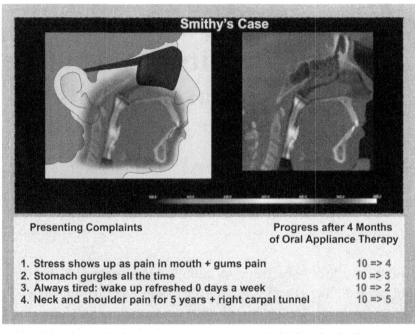

Smithy's Case

Presenting Complaints	Progress after 4 Months of Oral Appliance Therapy
1. Stress shows up as pain in mouth + gums pain	10 => 4
2. Stomach gurgles all the time	10 => 3
3. Always tired: wake up refreshed 0 days a week	10 => 2
4. Neck and shoulder pain for 5 years + right carpal tunnel	10 => 5

Color Scale: Red means a narrow airway with high risk of collapse during sleep; white means a wide airway with low risk.

Seven months after starting a particular type of oral-appliance therapy, Smithy reported that her Epworth Sleepiness Score had dropped from 14 to 9 and that she was sleeping better and dreaming more (a sign of deep sleep).

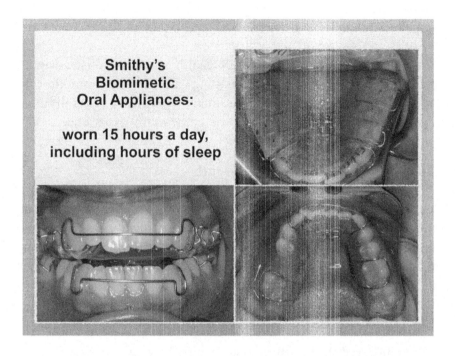

Smithy's
Biomimetic
Oral Appliances:

worn 15 hours a day,
including hours of sleep

Fourteen months later, her symptom score dropped 87 percent compared to pre-oral-appliance therapy. She admits that she works at a computer all day without good posture.

Symptoms	Before treatment	4 months later	14 months later
Pain in mouth and gums	10	4	0
Stomach gurgling	10	3	2
Always tired	10	2	0
Pain @ neck-shoulder-wrist	10	5	3
Symptom score	40	14	5

Smithy's case shows that the mouth structure plays a role in symptoms inside, around, and beyond the mouth. Note that Smithy had immaculate oral hygiene. She was just stuck with a structurally impaired mouth.

An impaired mouth hurts overall health while a Holistic Mouth promotes total health. Redeveloping an impaired mouth into a Holistic Mouth can improve many symptoms naturally and unexpectedly. This is a consistent outcome in my experience.

The High Cost of Missing the Mouth

Behind most puzzling medical, dental, and mood symptoms lurk an impaired mouth and a pinched airway. The problem is that the mouth is missing from the radar of 99.9 percent of health professionals today, judging from the experience of my new patients. This oversight has left many patients going from doctor to doctor for answers, often with very costly consequences. Here are few examples.

"They insisted that nothing was wrong." – G.A.'s Story

After she had gone to the emergency room complaining of dizziness and spent a whole day in testing at the adjoining hospital, G.A.'s health insurance carrier was handed a bill for over $11,000. "We didn't find anything wrong," said the doctors. "Here's a referral to a neurologist."

An amateur marathoner, G.A. was fit, trim, and happily semiretired in her mid-forties. Her best friend was a strong advocate of holistic health and referred her to me. The source of G.A.'s woes turned out to be a new filling. Her problem was solved for $350.

No one at her hospital ever looked in her mouth or asked about her dental history.

Even though the mouth and the body are connected, that's not the case in American health care today. There is a division between medical versus dental in both clinical care and health insurance that does not exist in the body. Dentists do teeth, doctors do body and mind, and the mouth is left off the body. In practice, this division can and does result in "missing mouth syndrome"—with serious consequences.

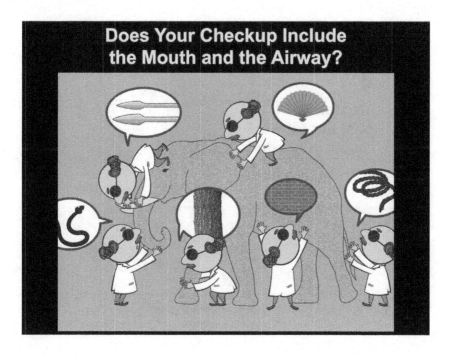

A Mouthful of Dental Trouble Is Connected to a Chartful of Medical Issues

T.D. had retired from a military career and gone to work for the federal government. His presenting complaints included erectile dysfunction, declining memory, teeth grinding, and intolerance of sleeping with a CPAP (continuous positive airway pressure) mask for sleep apnea. He had been diagnosed with obstructive sleep apnea (OSA), which comes with a host of ripple effects. Among them is acid reflux, which had eroded the inside two-thirds of his teeth.

T.D.'s dentists fixed his teeth as needed, and his doctors treated his sleep apnea according to the standard of care, but he was still left with the medical and dental aftermath of OSA-related complications. Because of this, T.D. could not even start to redevelop his jaws and airway. He was stopped cold by the more than $20,000 it would cost to restore his twenty-three acid-dissolved teeth to proper form and function with crowns so that they would be fit to anchor oral appliances.

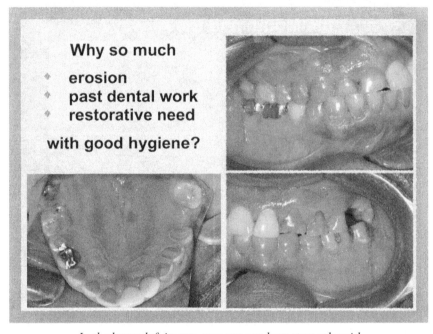

In the lower left image, you can see how stomach acid reflux has dissolved the inside of all teeth.

In my view, G.A., T.D., and all their attending doctors and dentists are victims of a health-care system that perpetuates medical, dental, and mental divisions that do not exist inside the body.

What Doctors Don't Know Hurts Them Too

Recognition of the mouth's role in total health is the first step toward effective solutions. My patients frequently ask me, "Why has no other doctor or dentist ever mentioned impaired mouth to me?" after learning that they had been stuck with an impaired mouth for years.

Many doctors of all specialties have admitted to me privately after my lectures on oral-systemic connections, "I try to look into my patients' mouths, but honestly I don't know what I am looking at."

Doctors and dentists themselves can suffer from impaired mouths just like their patients because Holistic Mouth is not part of their curriculum. Here are three cases:

- Dr. Y was a chiropractic doctor who had had neck pain and teeth grinding for as long as she could remember. Chiropractic adjustment would give short-term relief, but the pain always returned the next day. Within a half hour of putting on her bite-correction appliance, her pain was gone. Wearing it through the night, she actually feels refreshed now after sleeping.

- Dr. X was a medical doctor who worked fourteen to sixteen hours a day, took lots of supplements, and lived with neck and shoulder pain. She could control her food choices and meal portions, but not her snoring, teeth grinding, jaw clenching, and the resulting head, neck, and jaw pain. Her health was a constant struggle, mostly because her craniofacial and jaw structures were orthopedically misaligned.

- Dr. Z was an integrative medical doctor who found his three-tooth bridge on his pillow one morning—with roots attached! He had been medically diagnosed early with OSA, but his dentist did not know the connection between airway obstruction and teeth grinding, which I find to be a leading cause of tooth loss in patients with good oral hygiene. Dr. Z had lost twelve of his thirty-two teeth, and the remaining ones showed significant wear and tear.

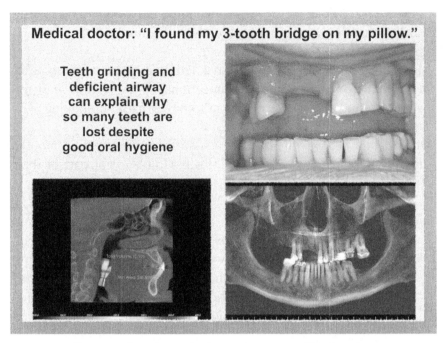

Medical doctor: "I found my 3-tooth bridge on my pillow."

Teeth grinding and deficient airway can explain why so many teeth are lost despite good oral hygiene

Green on the color scale does not mean good but less than ideal. White is ideal. "Sleep bruising" is the medical term for teeth grinding, which, in my opinion, is an airway issue.

How could patients know about these mouth-body connections if their doctors and dentists do not?

We have seen just a glimpse of what can happen to our overall health when the mouth is left off the body map. The traditional medical-dental divide has left many patients with an impaired mouth saddled with missed diagnoses, ineffective or incorrect treatment, and big bills. A more holistic view of how the whole body works is needed.

Integrating Mind-Body-Mouth to Turn On Natural Health

Seeing impaired mouth structure as a source of health troubles is still a very new idea in 2017, even though every patient knows that the mouth is connected to the body. WholeHealth is a "wholistic" way to seeing and integrating the body's various systems into a more functional and self-renewing whole. The science of oral-systemic links, and sleep medicine in particular, has led us to the new frontier of WholeHealth integration.

The earth is no longer flat, and adults are no longer stuck behind the proverbial eight ball of an impaired mouth and pinched airway. However, to successfully treat these conditions, health professionals must break down their "'silo mentality" and collaborate seamlessly for high-order health.

An Impaired Mouth comes with predictable consequences baked in, and a diverse set of symptoms will normalize when impaired mouth structures (as a root cause) are corrected. This principle holds regardless of technology or appliances, which will no doubt change with time.

The case outcomes presented in this book do not represent final proof; instead, they are early precedents of what is possible when impaired mouth syndrome is recognized and properly treated with Holistic Mouth solutions. I present them with great humility and deep respect for all the researchers, professors, mentors, and patients whose generous teaching and self-less sharing collectively help make the concept and practice of Holistic Mouth Solutions.

Holistic Mouth Bites

- Holistic Mouth is about the role of the mouth in whole body health. Consider getting a Holistic Mouth checkup when natural health goes wrong or does not come back.

- An impaired mouth is the start of a domino effect leading to and perpetuating pain, fatigue, and many diseases resistant to conventional treatment, but it is frequently overlooked in health care today.

- Behind most puzzling medical, dental, and mood symptoms lurk an impaired mouth and a pinched airway. Recognizing the mouth's role in total health can help solve many diverse symptoms at the causal level.

- Holistic Mouth Solutions is a WholeHealth approach to turn back illness and turn on wellness starting with the mouth's structural form for supporting overall health through not only food and drink, but also airway and sleep.

Chapter Two

Good Mouth, Bad Mouth

Oral diseases and conditions are associated with other health problems.

– Oral Health in America:
A Report of the Surgeon General [1]

"Holistic Mouth" is a term I coined to put the missing mouth back into whole-body health. The mouth and its owner-operator both play pivotal roles between illness and wellness. Total health has a better chance when the mouth can do all its health-supporting functions with the right form (structure).

What Is a Holistic Mouth? Why the State of Your Mouth Matters

A Holistic Mouth has a sufficiently developed structure to support whole-body health with these essential functions (ABCDES):

- **Alignment** of the head, jaws, and spine to alleviate pain, depression, and fatigue naturally

- **Breathing** without airway obstruction by tongue, day and night

- **Circulation** without dental infections or oxygen deficiency

- **Digestion** without ingesting toxins and causing inflammation

- **Emotional** to maintain or recover health and to feel good every day

- **Sleep** without airway obstruction, snoring, or teeth grinding

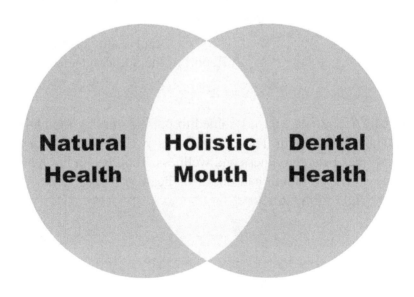

Holistic Mouth is about the role of the mouth in whole body health. One simple measure of a Holistic Mouth is whether you sleep well and wake up refreshed consistently. Another is how quickly you recover from illness, injury, or stress.

Mouth breathing, for example, allows bacteria and viruses to get in unchecked, whereas nasal breathing comes with the immune defense built in. Snoring and mouth breathing deprive the body of nitric oxide, a blood-vessel dilator (and the active ingredient for treating erectile dysfunction) made naturally from nasal breathing.

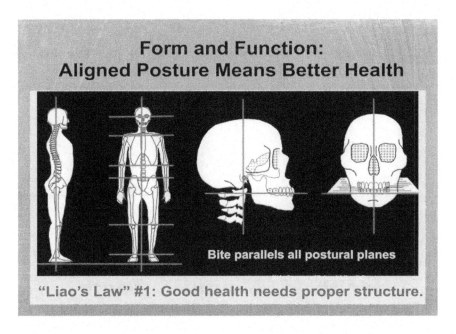

Form and Function:
Aligned Posture Means Better Health

Bite parallels all postural planes

"Liao's Law" #1: Good health needs proper structure.

How Your Impaired Mouth Can Harm Your Health

An impaired mouth interferes with the health of the whole body. An impaired mouth can eat, drink, talk, and even smile, but its poor form interferes with its other jobs of supporting ABCDES. An impaired mouth harms your overall health in three ways:

- **Poor mouth structure:** crowded/crooked teeth; bad bite patterns, such as a deep overbite, underbite, open bite, or crossbite; a tongue-tie; a weak chin; a long, narrow face or flat, wide face; and so on, all of which interfere with ABCDES and cause related health troubles

- **Poor mouth style:** misuse and overuse, as in having a sweet tooth or stress eating; neglect as in poor oral hygiene; and unhealthy habits, such as habitual mouth breathing, lip biting, fingernail or pencil chewing, tongue cushioning between the teeth, and tight-lipped swallowing that results in mouth wrinkles and "sad smile" lines around the mouth

- **Both**

America's health-care bills show that most mouths today are not only overused, but also structurally impaired.

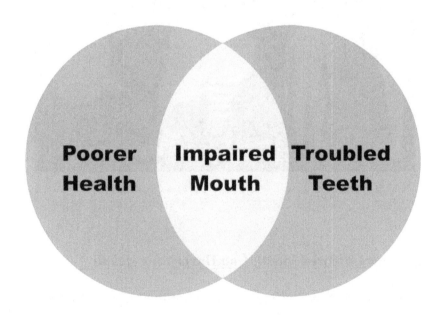

Frequent symptoms of an impaired mouth can include:

- Pain in the head, jaws, neck, shoulders, or back that persists despite treatment

- Chronic fatigue, depression, anxiety, excessive weight gain

- Snoring, tiredness upon waking up, daytime sleepiness

- Teeth grinding, jaw clenching, dental sensitivity to hot and cold

- Sweet tooth, bleeding gums, diabetes, brain fog

- High blood pressure, heart attacks, stroke, dry mouth from medications

- Increasingly crowded front teeth, mouth wrinkles forming "sad smile" lines

- Broken back teeth needing crowns, root canals, extractions, or implants

- Malocclusion: crowded/crooked teeth or mismatch of upper and lower jaws

Impaired Mouth Syndrome

A patient with impaired mouth can have a diverse set of medical, dental, and psycho-emotional symptoms called Impaired Mouth Syndrome. Different patients can have different combinations of the symptoms listed above, which are rarely integrated in medical, dental, or hospital assessments. For example, malocclusion has been linked to obstructive sleep apnea in a 2008 Japanese study. [2]

In 2017 America, sleep apnea patients do not get evaluated for malocclusion, nor do patients with bunched up teeth and underdeveloped jaws get evaluated for sleep apnea risk. This is the inevitable outcome of artificially dividing the body into parts and classifying treatment into medicine, dentistry, chiropractics, osteopathics, naturopathics, acupuncture, etc., when no such departmental lines exist inside the body.

WholeHealth is the holistic way of seeing symptoms as reactions to causes, and Impaired Mouth Syndrome is the collection of subjective symptoms connected to deficient jaw structure. Many symptoms go away naturally when impaired mouth structure is recognized and treated, as the case studies in this book will show.

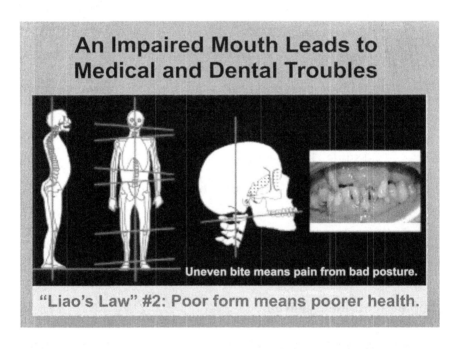

An Impaired Mouth Leads to Medical and Dental Troubles

Uneven bite means pain from bad posture.

"Liao's Law" #2: Poor form means poorer health.

Malocclusion: Why Dental and Skeletal Alignment Matters

A Holistic Mouth has good jaw structure, which means that there's bone volume for all teeth to align naturally and enough space between the jaws for the tongue to stay out of the throat.

Crowded teeth come from deficient jaws, which is a cardinal feature of impaired mouth. The bite—*occlusion* in dentistry—is where the upper and lower teeth come together. When they don't fit together peak-to-valley and/or when the jaws do not align with skull bones, we call it *malocclusion* (*mal-* means "bad" in Latin).

So malocclusion comes in two types: dental (teeth to teeth) and skeletal (jaw to jaw or jaw to skull). Dental occlusion refers to how upper and lower teeth fit into each other while skeletal malocclusion is the orthopedic (bone to bone) mismatch: How does the upper jaw fit into the head? How does the lower jaw fit into the upper?

Both dental and skeletal malocclusion come in three types—Class I, II, and III—named after the frequency of occurrence in the population. In general, Classes II and III are abnormal and often come with more medical and dental problems, but Class I is not immune.

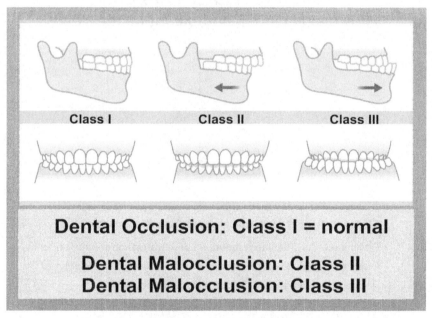

Drawing courtesy of Dr. Je-yang Jau of Taiwan

In my opinion, a dental malocclusion is secondary to a skeletal malocclusion diagnosis because skeletal malocclusion is a bigger source of the "three-foot cage." Skeletal malocclusion can affect dental occlusion, facial appearance, snoring, and sleep apnea.

Viewed from the side, a jaw is *protruded* when it is positioned forward relative to the forehead, as in gorillas or early humans. A jaw is *retruded* when it is positioned toward the back of the head. Weak chin and flat midface are features of an impaired mouth and frequent findings in patients with sleep, pain, and fatigue issues.

Because it has a greater effect on the airway, skeletal malocclusion should be treated *before* dental malocclusion. My patients find the following distinction useful: orthodontics (braces) treats dental malocclusion by moving teeth like boxcars on a railroad, whereas jaw orthopedics (oral appliances) develops rail beds to correct skeletal malocclusion.

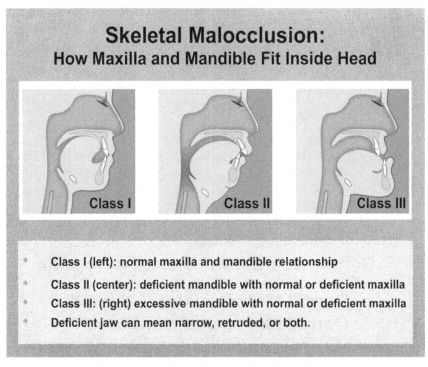

Skeletal Malocclusion:
How Maxilla and Mandible Fit Inside Head

Class I   Class II   Class III

- Class I (left): normal maxilla and mandible relationship
- Class II (center): deficient mandible with normal or deficient maxilla
- Class III: (right) excessive mandible with normal or deficient maxilla
- Deficient jaw can mean narrow, retruded, or both.

Illustration courtesy of Dr. Je-yang Jau of Taiwan

While crooked and/or crowded teeth are often a sign of malocclusion, perfectly straight teeth are not necessarily a sign of good occlusion. Straight teeth in skeletal malocclusion qualifies as impaired mouth.

I often see this type of "three-foot cage" in adults who had teeth extracted for braces in their teens. Symptoms of Impaired Mouth Syndrome, such as neck pain, jaw-joint clicks/pops/locks, snoring, sleep apnea, teeth grinding, and chronic fatigue are frequent in these patients.

"Life-Changing" Impaired-Mouth Correction: Sheila's Story

Sheila's jaw would lock up, and she had lots of neck and back pain when she woke up in the morning—"As if I'd been doing yard work all day." That was six years ago.

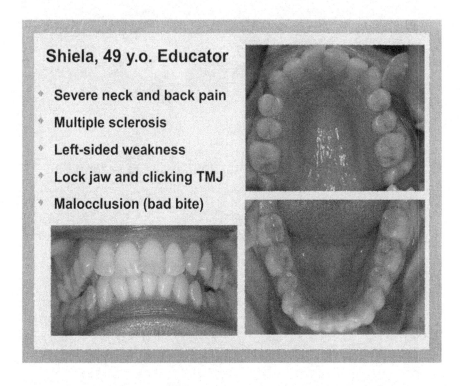

Shiela, 49 y.o. Educator
* Severe neck and back pain
* Multiple sclerosis
* Left-sided weakness
* Lock jaw and clicking TMJ
* Malocclusion (bad bite)

"I used to have MS (multiple sclerosis)," she says, "and now it's all behind me. The neck pain is now a 0 on a scale of 10, and I have no dental complaints. My energy is up, and I regained my balance after oral appliances corrected my bite and widened my palate. I started running again, which is huge for me. This has been life changing."

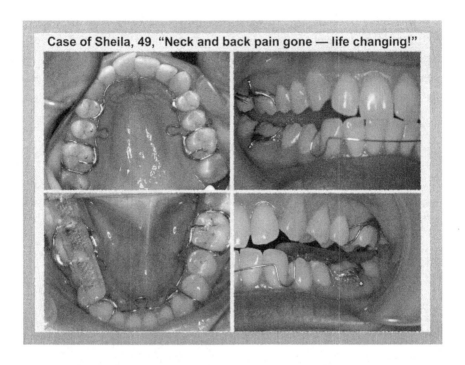

Case of Sheila, 49, "Neck and back pain gone — life changing!"

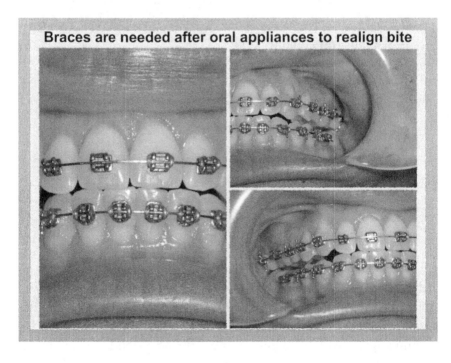

Braces are needed after oral appliances to realign bite

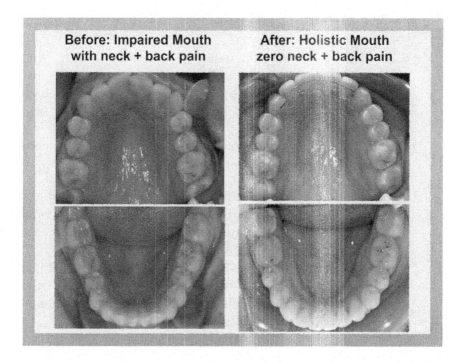

| Before: Impaired Mouth with neck + back pain | After: Holistic Mouth zero neck + back pain |

Sheila was a model patient, doing her part in treatment by wearing the appliances twelve to sixteen hours a day, seeing the recommended health professionals for necessary support, making the needed diet and lifestyle changes, and doing self-healing exercises. In my experience, most patients can comply with wearing oral appliances, but many slack off with integrative care and fail to sustain the necessary lifestyle changes.

Sheila's results are powerful proof of her commitment to following through.

Holistic Mouth Bites

- A Holistic Mouth facilitates whole-body health with alignment, breathing, circulation, digestion, energy, and sleep (ABCDES) while an impaired mouth interferes with ABCDES and blocks whole-body health.

- Can Sheila's "MS" happen be an overlap with Impaired Mouth Syndrome? I believe it is.

- Even though crooked, crowded teeth are often a sign of jaw underdevelopment, straight teeth inside jaws in skeletal malocclusion still constitute an impaired mouth.

- Straighten jaws before teeth because it has a greater effect on airway size, skeletal malocclusion of the jaws should be treated with oral appliances if possible before dental malocclusion is corrected with braces.

Chapter Three

Your Mouth-Body Connections: The Science of Oral-Systemic Links

Disease enters by mouth, and disaster exits by mouth.

– Chinese Proverb

Intuitively, we know that the mouth and body are connected. Now science has weighed in. Besides through nutrition and diet, the mouth can impact our overall health in many ways, including gum inflammation, sleep, snoring, sleep apnea, teeth grinding, mouth breathing, malocclusion (bad bite) and their related medical, dental, and mood symptoms.

Oral-Systemic Links is a growing compilation of scientifically established mouth-body connections that join the dental and medical spheres.

"Oral," of course, means the mouth, which is far more than just an opening in your head. It includes the upper and lower jaws that form two-thirds of the face, as well as the teeth, gums, jaws, jaw joints, muscles, tongue, tonsils, soft palate, ligaments, salivary glands, nerves, blood vessels, lips, skin over the jaws and face, and fascia, the fibrous and loose tissues under the skin and around and throughout all muscles, organs, and joints.

"Systemic," on the other hand, refers to the rest of the body: the brain, head, neck, spine, limbs, torso, internal organs, and all the physical tissues in, around, and between them, including bones, joints, muscles, fascia, blood, nerves, cells, and genes.

"Links" encompasses all the connections between the mouth and the whole body, including all systems governing posture, breath, circulation, digestion, and elimination—blood, lymph circulation, saliva, hormones, the immune system, neurotransmitters—*everything* that keeps the body functioning. The connections also include experience, memory, emotions, vital energy such as chi (*qi*), and the body's energetic meridians.

The Surprising Science That's Been Hiding in Plain Sight

Oral-systemic links are two-way phenomena. Mouth symptoms can have systemic causes, such as the left-sided jaw pain associated with angina and heart attack. Conversely, medical symptoms can have dental sources. Below are a few recent research findings that illustrate the mouth-body connections:

- A 2016 study in PLoS Medicine showed the link between *periodontitis* (gum disease) and memory decline: "The presence of periodontitis at baseline ... was associated with a six fold increase in the rate of cognitive decline." [1]

- Bacteria from the mouth have been shown to spread to the rest of the body. For instance, people with periodontal disease have double or triple the risk of having a heart attack or stroke, [2, 3]

- Oral bacteria have been found in heart-attack clots. "Dental infection and oral bacteria, especially viridans streptococci, may be associated with the development of acute coronary thrombosis," says a 2013 study in the journal *Circulation*.[4]

- The DNA from endodontic (root canal) bacteria was found in 56 percent of thirty-six samples of heart-attack clots in another 2013 study. Periodontal bacteria were found in 47 percent of those samples. The authors concluded that "dental infection could be part of pathophysiology in intracranial aneurysm disease [stroke]."[5]

- The mouth is where stress often shows up, according to one study published in *Brain Research*. Overeating may be a stress-driven reaction.[6]

- Sleep apnea has been shown to be a significant contributor to both Alzheimer's disease and diabetes.[7]

- A study in *Heart Failure Reviews* suggested that sleep apnea should be seen as "the new cardiovascular disease." [8]

In light of such evidence, leading doctors and integrative health professionals now recognize the mouth-body connection. In fact, in 2011, dentist Dr. Richard H. Nagelberg said, "The oral-systemic connections are accepted at this point by the medical and dental connections."[9]

"I am constantly amazed at how powerful a predictor of health your teeth are," says Dr. Joseph Mercola of Mercola.com. "When I have seen chronically ill patients with nearly cavity-free teeth, I am encouraged that they will likely get well quickly. If, on the other hand, their mouths are full of fillings and root canals, the prognosis is not as good." [10]

Dr. Jerry Tennant, the author of *Healing Is Voltage*, concurs: "Chronically ill patients need an informed dentist more than a medical doctor." [11]

The problem: while most people know that the mouth feeds the heart, the brain, and the body, and more and more doctors are aware of the perio-cardio connection, far fewer know about the impaired mouth-pinched airway connection. Naturopathic and chiropractic doctor Louisa Williams does:

> In my 30 years as a holistic physician specializing in dental issues, if a patient presents with a major malocclusion, then the treatment of this is truly sine qua non before (or at least in conjunction with) any other therapies. That is, positive dietary changes, nutritional supplementation, structural treatments (craniosacral therapy or spinal alignment), and even the most curative treatment—constitutional homeopathy—will never have a truly satisfying effect in the case of an impaired airway and the reduced oxygen delivery created 24/7 by a significant orofacial dysfunction. This issue must be addressed by an orthopedically trained biological dentist utilizing functional appliance therapy. [12]

The mouth-airway connection is even more foundational to health and survival than food and water, and oxygen level is a pivotal factor in chronic infections and periodontal-heart disease inflammation, in my opinion.

Mouth-Airway Connections

"Go to sleep" is the standard advice when you get a cold or come down with an illness. How fast you recover depends not only on the quantity but also the quality of your sleep. This is where having a wide-open airway is an asset and having an airway occupied by the tongue is a liability.

If the airway behind the soft palate and tongue is narrow, the risk of airway collapse goes up because an obstruction by the tongue creates a vacuum.

A narrow airway can be objectively documented with a 3-D cone-beam computed tomography (CBCT) scan: "3- dimensional CBCT airway analysis could be used as a tool to assess the presence and severity of OSA." [13]

A color scale is used to show the risk of airway collapse leading to obstructive sleep apnea. Red means high risk; white means low risk. Green is somewhere in the middle—not horrible, but hardly ideal.

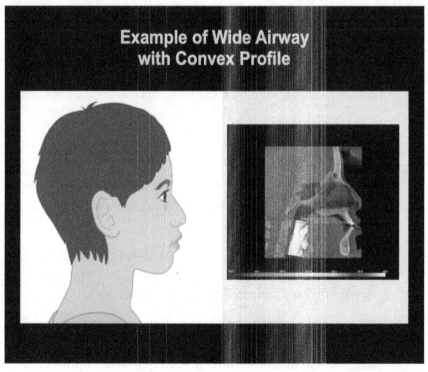

On the color scale, white means a uniformly wide airway with a low risk of airway collapse/obstruction; red means a high risk of collapse while black is off-the-chart dangerous.

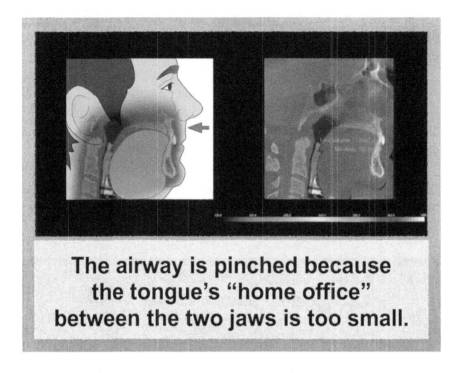

The airway is pinched because the tongue's "home office" between the two jaws is too small.

Holistic Mouth Bites

- Science has confirmed the oral-systemic links—an ever-increasing number of mouth-body connections that join the dental and medical spheres.

- Oral-systemic links are two-way streets. The whole can affect the mouth, and the mouth can have systemic-wide ripple effects. Thus medical symptoms can have oral sources.

- If the airway behind the soft palate and tongue is narrow, the risk of airway collapse goes up. Such oxygen deficiency leads to and magnifies a wide variety of health problems.

Chapter Four

Saving His Life & Her Sanity: "It's Like He's Strangling in His Sleep" (Case Study)

My husband has a sleep pattern that wakes him up from a seemingly sound sleep every twenty minutes almost in a panic. It's like he is strangling ... and it's concerning because its affecting both of our lives and how we feel the next day. We are more tired.

— Mrs. D.E.

There are all kinds of people but only two kinds of mouths. A Holistic Mouth promotes total health and facial radiance while an impaired mouth starts a cascade of medical, dental, mood, and financial troubles. In my experience, the troublemaker is very often an underdeveloped set of jaws that cannot accommodate the tongue between them.

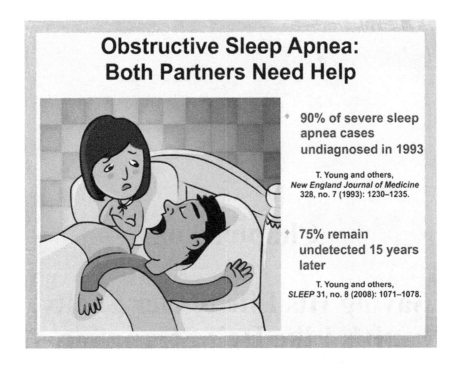

Saving a Marriage While Saving a Life: The Case of D.E.

D.E., a forty-seven-year old lawyer, was referred to me by his nutritionist. His presenting health complaints included:

> Pain in low back [L4/5] and mid-upper back, poor digestion and bloating, frequent sinus infections and bouts of congestion, heart arrhythmia sometimes, and a mouth that had always felt too small for his tongue.

It's worth noting that D.E.'s wife was concerned about his troubled breathing and her own sleep while D.E.'s focus was on his pain.

When he opened his mouth, I saw spotlessly clean teeth and gums. D.E. commented, "My dentists have never found anything wrong with me. But my nutritionist thinks my mouth may be the cause of my remaining health issues."

"Besides the symptoms you've mentioned, how is your day-to-day stress level on a scale of zero to ten?"

"I'd say six."

"How's your weight in relation to where you'd like to be?"

"I suffer from living the good life, with good wine and all the foods that go with it. But I work out regularly to keep the weight at bay."

"How many days a week do you wake up feeling refreshed?"

"Two. Maybe one."

"That can be a clue pointing to an impaired mouth. When was the last time you had a medical and dental checkup?"

"I see a chiropractor every two weeks to avoid medication and surgery, and I have my dental checkup and cleaning every six months without fail, so there's not much for them to do."

"What do they tell you about your symptoms?"

"Not much, other than come back every six months."

"Anything else you want to add?"

"I believe in the power of essential oils, alkaline water, nutrition, and massage. I do them all, but I seem to have hit a wall in my health quest."

"OK. Let's do our CSI: chair-side investigation. We'll start by connecting your posture with your bite, which can have a role in your chronic pain."

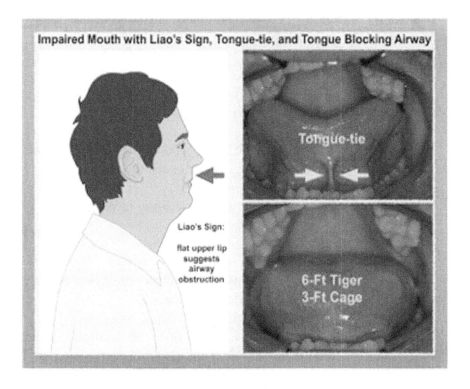

Impaired Mouth with Liao's Sign, Tongue-tie, and Tongue Blocking Airway

Tongue-tie

Liao's Sign:

flat upper lip
suggests
airway
obstruction

6-Ft Tiger
3-Ft Cage

The Importance of a Holistic Mouth Checkup: Is Your Mouth Hurting Your Health?

Imagine driving across the country in a high-end car with defective steering. The tires will wear out sooner, the trip will likely be unpleasant and costly, and the destination may be beyond reach.

The same is true with going through life with an impaired mouth, which "is much more than healthy teeth," as US Surgeon General Dr. David Satcher put it in *Oral Health in America*.[1] D.E.'s case shows what can happen to overall health when the mouth is structurally impaired, even if the teeth and gums are fine.

Holistic Mouth checkup for D.E. revealed a significantly impaired mouth with:

- A forward neck and backward head tilt that is typical of people with narrow airways

- Habitual mouth breathing from chronically stuffy nose

- Malocclusion with misaligned upper and lower dental midlines, which is a frequent source of neck, shoulder, and back pain

- A deep overbite (5 mm vs. the ideal of 1 to 2 mm) and retruded jaws, which combine to offer the normal size 6 tongue with a size 3 space

- Extraction of two upper premolars for orthodontics in high school, which had reduced his arch length and the oral volume for his tongue

- Tongue-tie anchoring his tongue to the floor of the mouth instead of its roof—a recipe for a deficient upper jaw and crowded teeth.[2] A tongue-tie is a short and tight ligament under the tongue that limits its movements and confines it to the floor of the mouth, which contributes to impaired mouth development— see chapter 13.

- An abnormal swallowing pattern involving a gurgling sound, coupled with forceful contractions of muscles around his mouth (In my opinion, this abnormal swallowing had contributed to the relapse of prior orthodontic treatment.)

- A very narrow airway (in the orange-red zone of color scale), highly susceptible to sleep apnea [3]

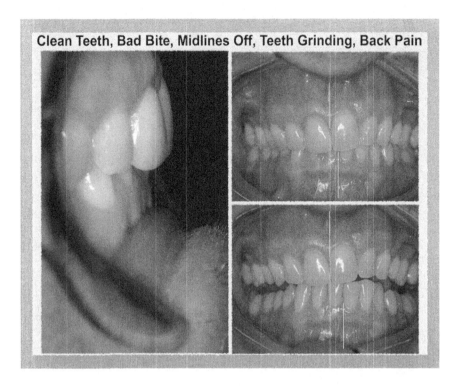

Clean Teeth, Bad Bite, Midlines Off, Teeth Grinding, Back Pain

The mouth, in side view, is convex and full when an airway is wide, which I see only once in a blue moon. In profile, D.E.'s upper lip was flat.

Now look at the young lady in the image below, and imagine squashing her upper and lower jaw and its contents into her face, toward the back of the head. That is exactly how an impaired mouth pinches the airway.

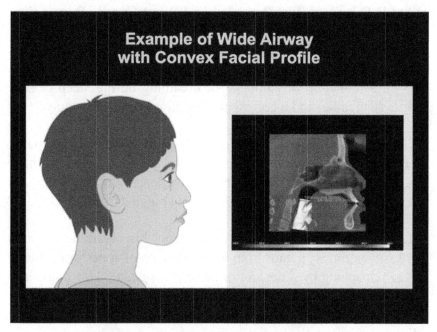

Example of Wide Airway with Convex Facial Profile

On the color scale, white end means low risk of airway collapse, red means a high risk, and black is off-the-chart dangerous.

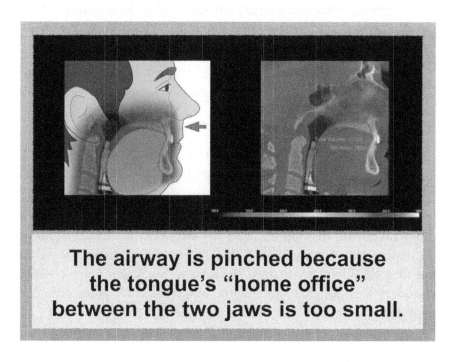

The airway is pinched because the tongue's "home office" between the two jaws is too small.

What D.E.'s Sleep Test Revealed and What Can Be Done

Suspecting a pinched airway inside an impaired mouth, I sent D.E. for a sleep test, which confirmed severe obstructive sleep apnea (OSA), a reduction or stoppage of breathing during sleep despite efforts to breathe, and a corresponding drop in oxygen supply.[4]

To experience an apnea event, try this: Inhale and exhale normally, then cover your nose and mouth with your hands so no air gets in or out as you count "one, one thousand; two, one thousand" until you get to eleven. Now lift your hand. Aren't you glad to get that breath?

D.E.'s sleep test showed that, on average, his breathing suffered thirty-seven times an hour from a combination of apnea or his blood oxygen dropping by 4 percent or more (*hypopnea*)! This number—the apnea-hypopnea index (AHI)—is often used as a benchmark for OSA. Here's how the results break down, according to the Cleveland Clinic's online medical reference:

> **Mild OSA:** *AHI of 5–15.* Involuntary sleepiness during activities that require *little* attention, such as watching TV or reading
>
> **Moderate OSA:** *AHI of 15–30.* Involuntary sleepiness during activities that require *some* attention, such as meetings or presentations
>
> **Severe OSA:** *AHI of more than 30.* Involuntary sleepiness during activities that require *more active* attention, such as talking or driving[5]

After reviewing his options with his sleep-test doctor, D.E. chose oral-appliance therapy over CPAP, which is a mask worn over the face that delivers air past the airway blockage under positive pressure. Besides, his chief complaint was back pain, and oral appliance can fix pain.

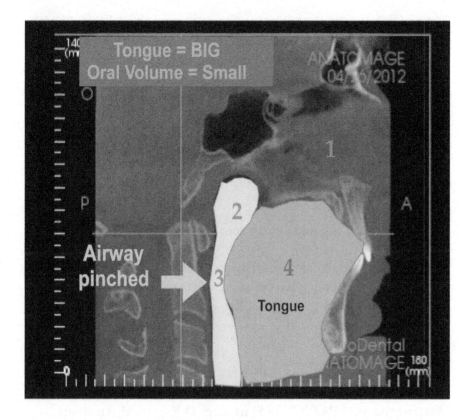

"The three-foot cage makes sense now," D.E. said. He pointed to the orange bulge on his CT image above. "That whole thing is the tongue? I had no idea it's that huge! It's a wonder I'm alive and can get any work done."

"It is indeed. And there are more health hazards ahead if it's left untreated."

"That's why I'm here. Is there any hope for me?"

"Yes, thanks to the new science of epigenetics and the new breed of oral appliances that can switch on your genes to increase your jaw size as if you were a teenager again to regrow and realign your jaws to fix pain naturally."

"Sounds good. What else do I need to know?"

"In my practice, oral appliances are just one part of WholeHealth-oriented Holistic Mouth Solutions. In your case, we'd first have you do the oral-appliance therapy plus myofunctional therapy (chapter 13) to retrain your mouth to swallow correctly—after your tongue-tie is released and your diet tweaked to minimize stuffy nose.

"In phase 2, you'll wear orthodontics to bring your teeth back into a stable peak-to-valley bite. Finally, we'll do some restorative dentistry to replace those two upper teeth that were extracted for braces."

"Now I see why my nutritionist sent me here. I'm in. Let's do it."

"You should know that phase 1 takes about a year in mild cases. In severe cases like yours, two or more years is common. Phase 2 can take sixteen to twenty-four months, depending on case complexity and patient compliance."

"I can't wait to get started."

Alternative to CPAP's Life Sentence: D.E.'s Oral-Appliance Therapy

Oral appliances are custom-made mouthpieces worn over the teeth to free the body from the tyranny of an impaired mouth with its bad bite and pinched airway. They come in many types. D.E.'s set of oral appliances was designed to relieve his whole body of his bad bite and to widen his airway during sleep.

Treatment: Oral Appliances 16 Hours a Day and Oral Face Mask Worn During Sleep

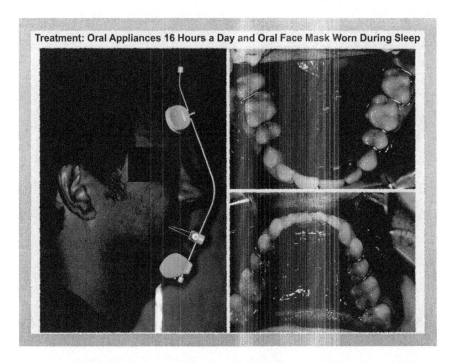

D.E.'s Initial Oral Appliances to Make Room for His Tongue

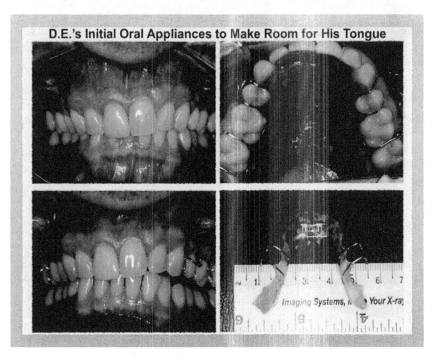

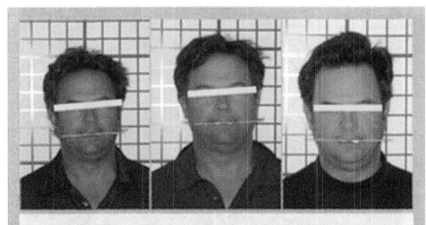

Leveling the maxilla with oral appliances as part of holistic mouth solutions takes away his back pain.

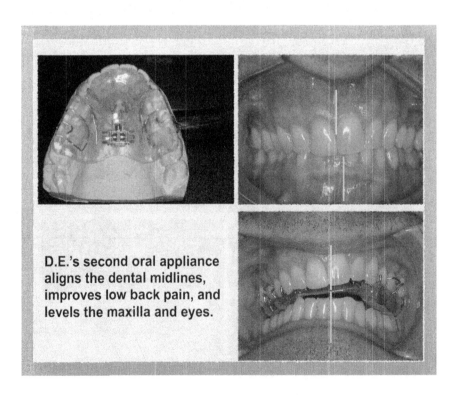

D.E.'s second oral appliance aligns the dental midlines, improves low back pain, and levels the maxilla and eyes.

"Huge Improvement" That Typical Doctors and Health Professionals Can't Touch

D.E.'s symptoms improved quickly after starting oral-appliance therapy. He faithfully followed my prescribed Holistic Mouth Solutions, which included acupuncture and osteopathic care, going to bed by 11:00 p.m., and continuing his chiropractic visits and sound nutrition.

Two months after we began, his airway had improved by 56 percent. At three and a half months, he had this to say:

> I came to Dr. Liao suffering from back pain for most of my life. I have seen chiropractic doctors and nutritionists but never saw any real relief. Now, after wearing an oral appliance, my airway has opened up 70% and my low back pain is almost nonexistent.

After fifteen months, he reported that his blood pressure had "gone down quite a bit: from 140/90 to 110/60 now. So it's been a huge improvement—I feel so much calmer."

I find that unexpected symptom improvements are common in patients undergoing oral-appliance therapy. It had not even occurred to D.E. that he had lived with anxiety until it went away with oral appliances that opened his airway as he slept.

Two years later, "Blood pressure, weight, wellness, ability, breathing all good," he reported. "Breathing is easier, and tongue fits better into upper mouth. And by the way, I won the tennis tournament at my club without having to use knee and back braces."

D.E.'s subjective improvement was documented in his systemic evaluations as well. One month after starting oral-appliance therapy, D.E.'s nutritional therapist sent his EAV (electro-acupuncture according to Voll) report (see below), showing that the body burden was much less. (In these images, green is good; red and yellow are not.)

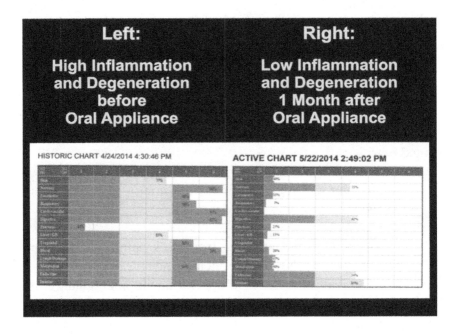

Ten months later, another report showed that D.E. was systemically "cleaner" and that his body had regained the ability to respond to nutritional therapy quickly.

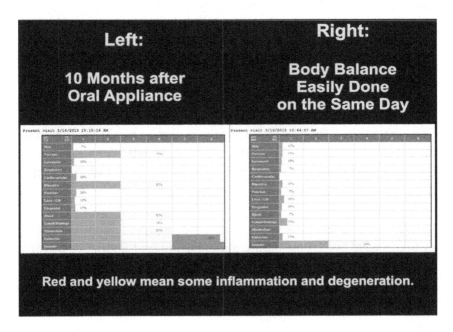

Oral-appliance therapy helped make this progress possible by turning D.E.'s impaired mouth around toward a Holistic Mouth.

Holistic Mouth Bites

- A clean dental bill of health does not mean the mouth is trouble-free. Evaluating the state of the airway and seeing the size 6 tiger tongue inside a size 3 mouth can provide clues.

- Living with an impaired mouth amounts to driving a top-end car with a broken wheel. The journey is bumpier and costlier, and the quest for health feels beyond reach.

- An impaired mouth is no longer a life sentence. Wearing oral appliances to sleep is simple, and positive outcomes are predictable with patient cooperation.

Chapter Five

CSI for Your Mouth: Revealing the Secrets of an Impaired Mouth Detective

Awareness is prerequisite to all acceptable changes of theory.

– Thomas S. Kuhn,
The Structure of Scientific Revolutions[1]

Sleeping with a tongue that closes your airway and threatens your life amounts to a dry form of waterboarding night after night. Signs of airway struggle can and often do show up in the mouth long before health slides downhill too far.

"CSI" in this book stands for "chair-side investigation", as mentioned earlier. With one look at a patient's face, I can often tell if they are at risk for an obstructed airway. You, too, can acquire Sherlock Holmes' eyes for recognizing an impaired mouth.

Postural Clues Pointing to a Pinched Airway

The first clue to an impaired mouth can be the posture of the head and neck in profile. In response to a pinched airway, the neck will extend forward, and the head may tilt backward in an effort to get more air. If you were to lie down in this posture, you'd be in the recommended posture for receiving CPR—neck extended, head back, and chin up.

This postural compensation eventually leads to a humped upper back and pain and/or stiffness in the neck and shoulders.

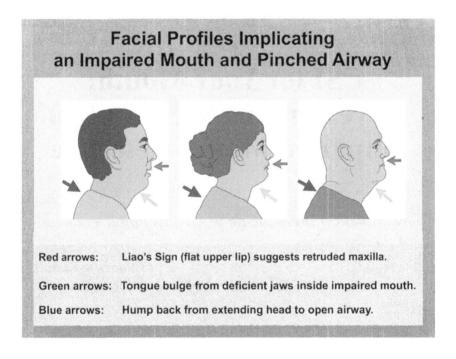

Facial Profiles Implicating an Impaired Mouth and Pinched Airway

Red arrows: Liao's Sign (flat upper lip) suggests retruded maxilla.

Green arrows: Tongue bulge from deficient jaws inside impaired mouth.

Blue arrows: Hump back from extending head to open airway.

Liao's Sign: CSI Clue #1

A flat or curled upper lip in profile view is such a regular feature in patients with an impaired mouth that I gave it a name: Liao's Sign.

Liao's Sign is a "rule of thumb" facial indicator of a retruded upper jaw that characterizes an impaired mouth. *Retrusion* is the opposite of protrusion. A retruded maxilla frequently results in a narrower airway behind the soft palate.

A positive Liao's Sign implicates a less-than-optimal airway until proven otherwise, yet the absence of Liao's Sign does not mean all is well. A non-retruded maxilla can still be too narrow, thus contributing to a three-foot cage.

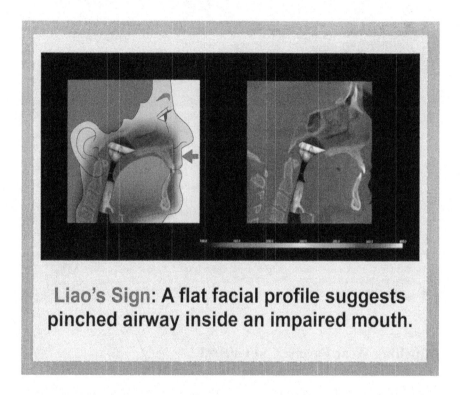

Liao's Sign: A flat facial profile suggests pinched airway inside an impaired mouth.

Friedman Tongue Position: CSI Clue #2

For predicting OSA in the absence of a CT scan, the position of the tongue at rest is a useful indicator. The Friedman Tongue Position (FTP) score is done with the mouth open and the tongue inside the lower dental arch.

The less you can see of the uvula (the tissue that hangs at the back of your mouth, above your throat), tonsils, and soft palate, the higher the risk of severe OSA, according to a 2011 Spanish study[2].

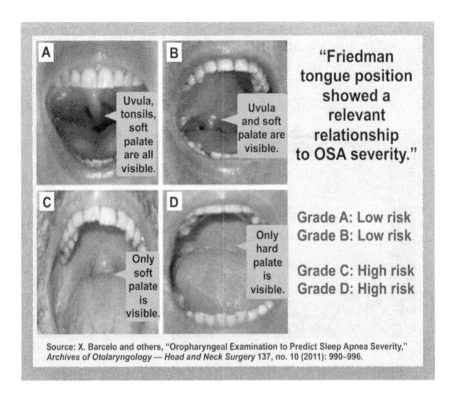

Source: X. Barcelo and others, "Oropharyngeal Examination to Predict Sleep Apnea Severity," *Archives of Otolaryngology — Head and Neck Surgery* 137, no. 10 (2011): 990–996.

Matching Wear Facets: CSI Clue #3

Matching wear facets between upper and lower teeth suggest teeth grinding, which in turn is connected to airway distress during sleep, as we shall see in Book 2.

Wear facets in molars tend to break teeth and loosen dental work while wear facets in front teeth can disfigure a pleasing smile. A sure way to look older than your age is to grind short your smile teeth. The next slide shows a normal bite and an unworn set of front teeth.

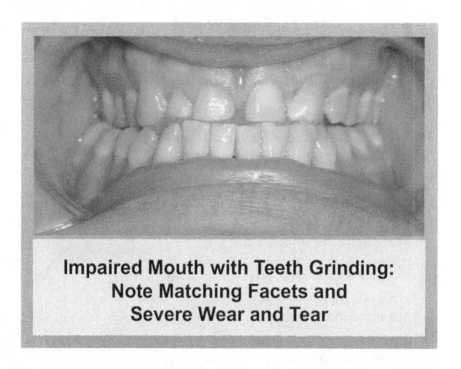

**Impaired Mouth with Teeth Grinding:
Note Matching Facets and
Severe Wear and Tear**

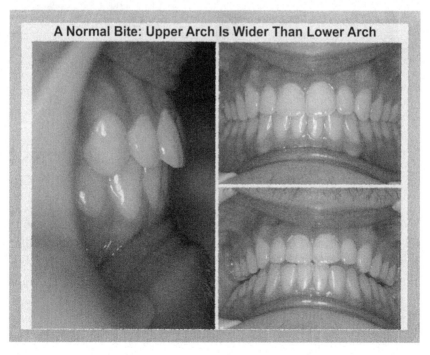

A Normal Bite: Upper Arch Is Wider Than Lower Arch

Malocclusion in Any Form: CSI Clue #4

In general, teeth crowding is a sign of malocclusion (bad bite), which can come from deficient jaws, which in turn is a frequent red flag for airway issues.

Straight teeth do not necessarily mean absence of malocclusion. For instance, a retruded maxilla with orthodontically straightened teeth is still a health liability.

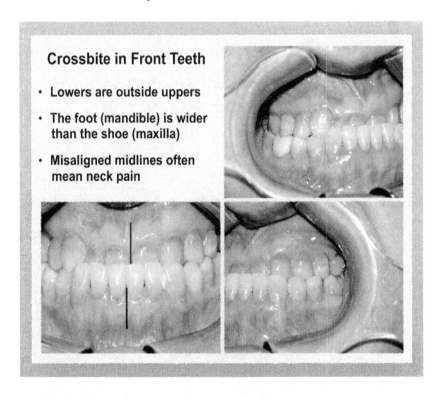

Crossbite in Front Teeth

- Lowers are outside uppers
- The foot (mandible) is wider than the shoe (maxilla)
- Misaligned midlines often mean neck pain

Malocclusion comes in many variations. A *crossbite* means one or more lower teeth lie outside the upper arch with teeth close together. Normally, the upper jaw should be wider than the lower. Crossbite suggests that the upper jaw is deficient in size or retruded in position.

Excessive Overbite and Overjet: CSI Clue #5

Two frequently used terms in malocclusion are *overbite* and *overjet*. "Overbite" refers to the vertical overlap between the upper and lower front teeth while "overjet" refers to the horizontal distance between upper and lower front teeth. In both cases, the ideal measure is 1 to 2 mm. Anything greater than this may indicate structural deficiency or imbalance.

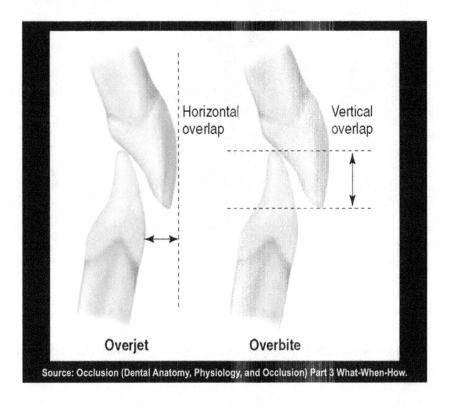

Source: Occlusion (Dental Anatomy, Physiology, and Occlusion) Part 3 What-When-How.

A deep overbite means that the ceiling of the tongue's habitat is very low, which implicates a pinched airway. Facially, a pronounced groove between the chin and the lower lip suggests a deep overbite.

The larger the overjet ("underbite"), the closer the lower jaw is to the throat, and the more the tongue is in the airway.

Weak chin is the surface sign of a large overjet and a retruded lower jaw below the surface dragging the tongue into the airway. Research from Japan has shown that "overjet was associated with the severity of obstructive sleep apnea syndrome in non-obese patients."[3]

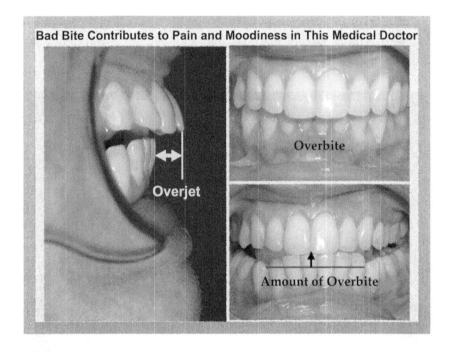

Bad Bite Contributes to Pain and Moodiness in This Medical Doctor

Overjet

Overbite

Amount of Overbite

Other Common Orofacial Clues to an Impaired Mouth

Other *orofacial* (mouth and face) signs indicating that all is not well with the mouth and airway can include:

Tooth prints on the sides of the tongue—medically called *crenation*—can mean poorer sleep. Research has found tongue scalloping to be predictive of sleep pathology.

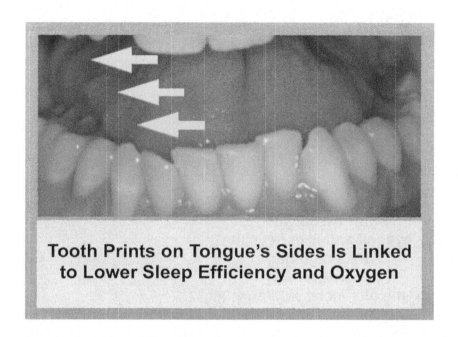

Tooth Prints on Tongue's Sides Is Linked to Lower Sleep Efficiency and Oxygen

Abfractions are notches of missing tooth structure at the gum line, which science has confirmed may be caused by teeth grinding. [4, 5] Abfractions are often very sensitive to cold and brushing.

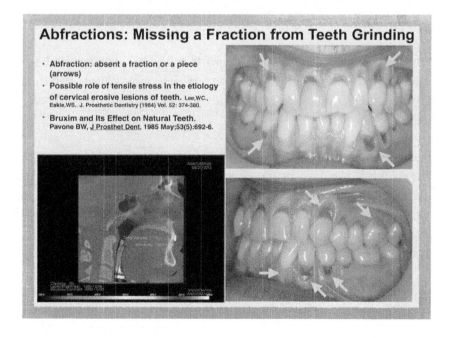

Abfractions: Missing a Fraction from Teeth Grinding

- Abfraction: absent a fraction or a piece (arrows)
- Possible role of tensile stress in the etiology of cervical erosive lesions of teeth. Lee,WC., Eakle,WS.. J. Prosthetic Dentistry (1984) Vol. 52: 374-380.
- Bruxim and Its Effect on Natural Teeth. Pavone BW, J Prosthet Dent, 1985 May;53(5):692-6.

Visible Sclera: Sclera is the white part of the eyeball. When sclera is visible between the lower eyelids and iris (the colored part of the eyes), it suggests a deficient maxilla (upper jaw) because the floor of the eyes is the roof of the maxilla.

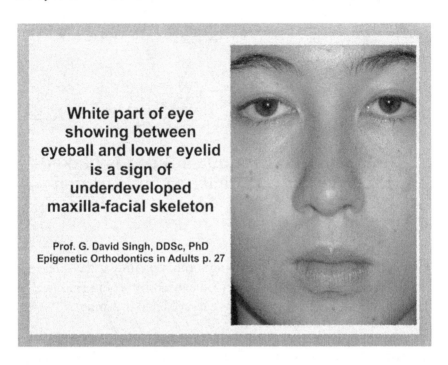

White part of eye showing between eyeball and lower eyelid is a sign of underdeveloped maxilla-facial skeleton

Prof. G. David Singh, DDSc, PhD
Epigenetic Orthodontics in Adults p. 27

Narrow nostrils and a small mouth with dry or chapped lips indicate chronic mouth breathing, which can cause abnormal craniofacial development. Both are visible in the image directly above.

Tori are bony outgrowths on the roof of the mouth, the tongue side of the lower jaw, or the cheek side of either jaw. They are the jawbone's response to excessive pressure from jaw clenching or teeth grinding. "In adults, it is likely that palatal and mandibular tori are manifestations of undiagnosed sleep-disordered breathing."[6]

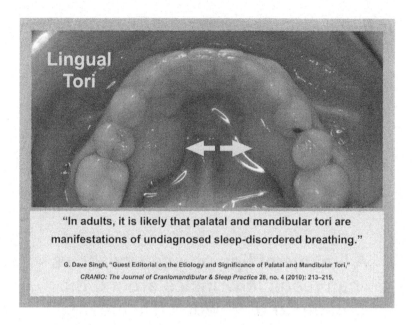

"In adults, it is likely that palatal and mandibular tori are manifestations of undiagnosed sleep-disordered breathing."

G. Dave Singh, "Guest Editorial on the Etiology and Significance of Palatal and Mandibular Tori," CRANIO: The Journal of Craniomandibular & Sleep Practice 28, no. 4 (2010): 213–215,

Facial creases and wrinkles around the mouth are more than a mere cosmetic issue. These deep creases and wrinkles come from a lifetime of improper swallowing. Keep in mind that you swallow a minimum of 1,000 times a day! Such improper swallowing can carve creases and etch wrinkles around the mouth over a lifetime.

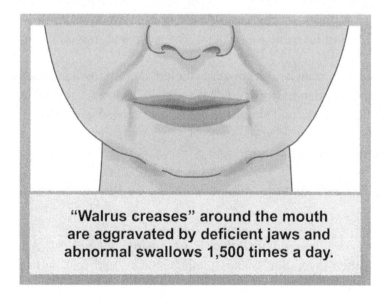

"Walrus creases" around the mouth are aggravated by deficient jaws and abnormal swallows 1,500 times a day.

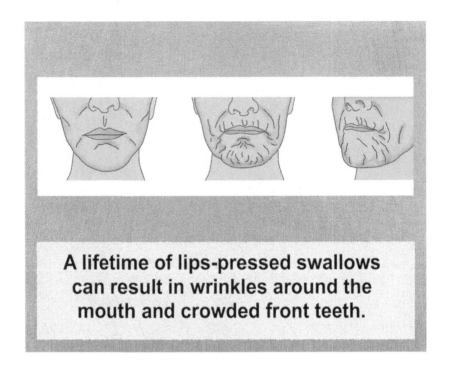

A lifetime of lips-pressed swallows can result in wrinkles around the mouth and crowded front teeth.

Beyond the Expertise of Dental Specialists: Dr. A's CSI

"I was a dentist in my country in South America," said Dr. A., a slim, trim, thirty-three-year-old stay-at-home mom with three kids. "But I fell in love and married an American and moved to DC."

Her list of current health concerns included brain fog and moodiness; low energy; depression and feeling sick in an indescribable way; achy head, neck, and shoulder; teeth that were sensitive to cold and sweets; teeth that felt rough and chalky; and a very dry mouth with an acidic taste in the morning.

"That's a lot to put up with while caring for three kids, Dr. Mom," I said.

"Yes, and I am worried that I am losing enamel." (Enamel is the surface layer that makes teeth beautiful and resistant to food abrasion.)

"Yes, you might be losing enamel to acid reflux. Please tell me about your medical history."

"I had lymphoma four years ago while I was pregnant with my first child. It was treated with chemo and radiation, and I've had two more kids since."

"You're a walking miracle!", I replied. "How many mornings a week do you wake up feeling refreshed?"

"I can't remember a good night's sleep in more than four years now. I wake up four to eight times every night because of the kids. The youngest is now one and a half."

"Amazing. I don't know how you do it." I added, "Did you have acid reflux before having children?"

"I used to have heartburn four years ago but not now—except when I cheat on my diet."

"Overall, what would you say is your biggest health issue?"

"I feel I have no energy in my tank to perform my job as a mom."

"You have a weak chin from a large (5 mm) overjet. Your tongue is like a six-foot tiger inside a three-foot cage formed by your jaws. This leads to a choke zone in your airway. Many of your symptoms are related to airway obstruction, including acid reflux and rough enamel from acid erosion. We'll need a sleep test to confirm."

"This is beginning to make sense now," said Dr. A. "My best friends back in my home country are dying to help me with their specialty. One is an oral surgeon who wants to do surgery, and the other is an orthodontist who wants to do braces for me. I know they mean well, but I'm glad I didn't let them do their thing on me."

"A wide-open airway is the real prize in the care of health. Let me share with you what I see in this photo of you standing in profile.

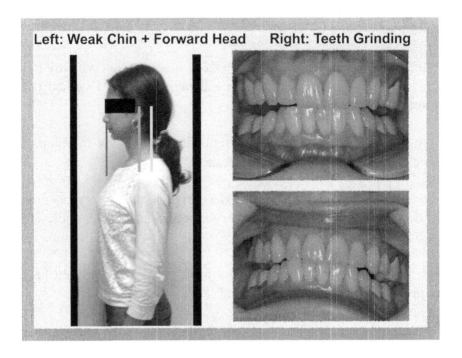

Left: Weak Chin + Forward Head   Right: Teeth Grinding

"Your head is forward with your ear opening—the green line—well ahead of your shoulder point, where the yellow line is. That's why you have head, neck, and shoulder pain.

"Your chin is weak, well behind the upper lip, which drives your tongue into your throat. That makes you susceptible to snoring, teeth grinding, dental sensitivity, jaw-joint clicks/pops/locks, and fatigue.

"Your upper front teeth are naturally straight and your smile is nice, but your upper arch is too narrow for your lower jaw. Moreover, you are likely to have wrinkles around your mouth as you get older because you swallow with your lips pressed together 1,500 times a day."

"No way are wrinkles around the mouth acceptable! I am glad you tell me that now. What else?"

"How many of these symptoms [in the next slide] do you have?" I asked Dr. A.

"That's me! We sure didn't learn this in dental school."

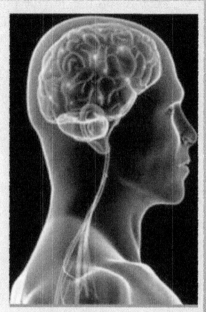

Teeth Grinders Often Suffer These Symptoms:

* Dental sensitivities
* Gum recession, broken teeth
* Sore jaws, clicking jaw joints
* Bladder urgency
* Morning headaches
* Daytime sleepiness
* Body aches and pains
* Brain fog, poor memory
* Depression, moodiness
* Chronic fatigue, adrenal exhaustion
* High blood pressure
* Higher dental and medical bills

Oxygen deficiency from airway obstruction is why.

"You're not alone, Dr. A. Dental schools train dentists to fix and save teeth, which serves an important basic need. But we're now in the new era of sleep medicine and oral-systemic links. So welcome to Holistic Mouth Solutions!"

"I can see some hope now."

Holistic Mouth Bites

- Seen through trained eyes, signs of airway struggle often show up in the mouth long before health slides downhill too far.

- Posture, profile, tongue position, occlusion, and features on the face and inside the mouth all provide clues to airway struggle in the absence of 3D CT imaging.

- A wide-open airway is the real prize in the care of health.

Chapter Six

The Damaging Domino Effect from an Impaired Mouth and Pinched Airway

Underdeveloped faces may indicate a collapse or constriction of the upper pharyngeal airway space.

– G. Dave Singh, DDSc, PhD, BDS,
Epigenetic Orthodontics in Adults[1]

Airway dictates, and the rest of the body accommodates. A human body can go for days without eating, but a brain does not last more than four minutes without oxygen. Oxygen on demand is a prerequisite for health and well-being. Just watch a baby sleep after a good feeding.

A good night's sleep is built on the foundation of a wide-open airway without choke points. Sleeping with a tiger tongue crowding the airway results in oxygen interruption during sleep threatens survival and elicits an involuntary response, which can include jaw clenching, teeth grinding, tossing and turning, elbowing and kicking, chest heaving, waking up with a gasp, bladder urgency, and a racing heart. You may or may not remember your airway struggle during sleep, but you will feel it the next morning in your mind, body, and mouth.

Repeating this pattern night after night will eventually lead to degeneration and health troubles. An impaired mouth structure is the first piece to fall in that domino. Let's take a closer look at the tongue inside the "three-foot cage" as it relates to the airway.

How a Tongue Becomes a Life-Threatening Tiger inside an Impaired Mouth

The tongue is fully functional at birth for feeding. This is a survival necessity. From then on, daily multitasking keeps the tongue fit through talking, eating, and swallowing saliva 1,200 times a day. So unlike the jaws, the tongue is never underdeveloped.

By contrast, the jaws and face take fifteen to eighteen years to reach final adult size and form. This is a long time in which craniofacial development can go wrong, including tongue-tie, a pathological swallow pattern (from bottle-feeding and long-term pacifier use), nutritional excess (junk foods) and deficiency (such as minerals for building bone), and habitual mouth breathing from chronic stuffy nose, among others. Many adults with sleep apnea, snoring, teeth grinding, and mood disorders have these signs and symptoms.

Anatomically, the back of the mouth merges with the upper airway—the *pharynx* that is between the back end of the nasal passage and the *trachea* (windpipe). In the slide below, Zone 1 is the nasal cavity while Zone 4 is the oral cavity, where the tongue belongs.

The *oral pharynx* is the space behind the tongue (Zone 3) while the *nasal pharynx* is the space (Zone 2) behind the soft palate at the back end of the upper jaw.

Upper Airway Spaces

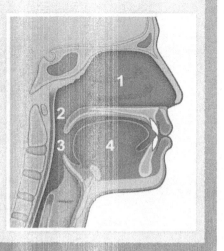

- **Zone 1: Nasal cavity**

- **Zone 2: Nasal pharynx**

- **Zone 3: Oral pharynx**

- **Zone 4: Oral cavity**

Good airway needs good form: ALL four zones wide and open.

In a Holistic Mouth, all four zones are wide open for uninterrupted oxygen delivery 24/7. So what might close them?

Structural defects have been linked to bony and tissue abnormalities, reports a 1997 study from Japan comparing the upper airway of sleep apnea and normal patients.[2] These load the pharynx and predispose it to airflow obstruction during sleep. These abnormalities can include:

- An oversized tongue (*macroglossia*)

- An undersized space ("three-foot cage") for the tongue

- Obesity around the jaws and neck

- Any combination of the above

This is worth repeating: the tongue belongs in the mouth, not the airway. When the tongue invades the airway and cuts oxygen delivery, the body reacts with distress—as if it is confronting a six-foot tiger threatening its life. Whether severe or mild, oxygen deficiency sets off a chain reaction throughout the body.

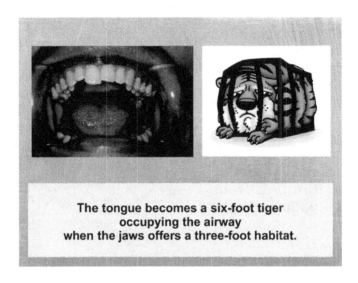

The tongue becomes a six-foot tiger occupying the airway when the jaws offers a three-foot habitat.

In my experience, adults with sleep apnea and teeth grinding frequently have a pinched airway inside an impaired mouth, and vice versa. Simply put:

Impaired Mouth = Pinched Airway = Medical, Dental, Mood Symptoms from Impaired Mouth Domino

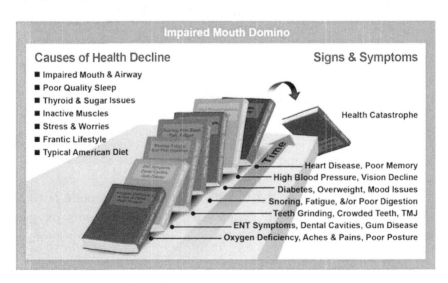

There is one important exception to the "normal size 6" tongue: swelling from hypothyroid (low) function, which is extremely common in the U.S.

A Super-Sized Tongue Is Linked to Hypothyroid, Pain, and Inflammation

In some cases, the tongue may be swollen, too large in and of itself. This may be caused by poor digestion or fluid retention, but among my patients, the most usual cause is hypothyroidism. Common signs of low thyroid function include cold hands and feet, a thin or missing outer third of the eyebrows, excess weight, thinning hair, and a hoarse voice.

Thyroid function is critically connected to both oral and total health. A 2014 study in the *Journal of Oral and Maxillofacial Pathology* reported: "The oral cavity is adversely affected by either an excess or deficiency of thyroid hormone. Childhood hypothyroidism known as cretinism is characterized by thick lips, large protruding tongue (macroglossia), malocclusion, and delayed eruption of teeth."[3]

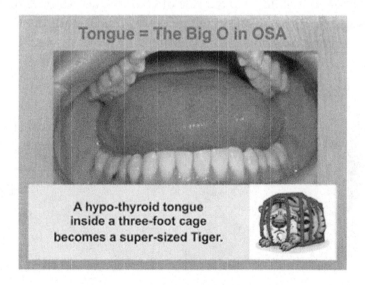

Tongue = The Big O in OSA

A hypo-thyroid tongue inside a three-foot cage becomes a super-sized Tiger.

In my experience, patients with thyroid disorders often have adrenal exhaustion from restless sleep night after night. They also have tighter muscles, tendons, and ligaments and more aches and pains. "Muscular dysfunction and tension resulting from hypothyroidism were major underlying factors in the development of TMJ syndrome … due to the increased incidence of jaw muscle spasm, muscular tension, and pain that are often associated with hypothyroidism," writes Dr. Mark Starr in *Hypothyroidism Type 2: The Epidemic*.[4]

This means hypothyroid patients can expect more creaky messages from their mouth and body when they start oral-appliance therapy. That's why, when I see a swollen tongue, I routinely refer my patient for a medical evaluation to rule out low thyroid function and to adjust the supplements as needed under medical supervision. This is WholeHealth integration.

Hypothyroid Tongue Test

Here's a simple test to see if you may be suffering from low thyroid: Stick out your tongue past your lips and check for space between the corners of your mouth and the side of your tongue. Absence of space suggests hypothyroidism -- I learned this from Dr. Jorge D. Flechas, MD, of Hendersonville, North Carolina.

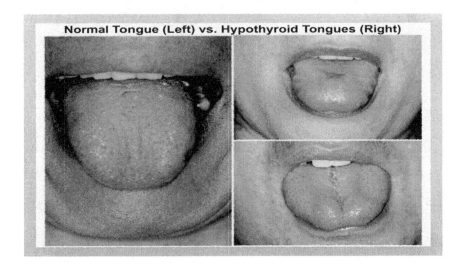

Normal Tongue (Left) vs. Hypothyroid Tongues (Right)

Inflammation goes down with treatment of hypothyroidism. For instance, a 2015 Brazilian study "observed significant changes in the inflammatory profile in hypothyroid patients under treatment, with reduction of pro-inflammatory cytokines and elevation of anti-inflammatory cytokine. In these patients, a decrease in low-grade chronic inflammation may have clinical relevance due to the known connection between chronic inflammation, atherosclerosis, and cardiovascular events."[5]

Treating hypothyroid properly works synergistically with oral appliances to reduce pain, fatigue, and heart disease. This is the WholeHealth part of Holistic Mouth Solutions.

Holistic Mouth Bites

- Airway dictates, and the rest of the body accommodates. This is "Rule 1" in how the body works.

- The tongue belongs in the mouth, not the airway. When the tongue occupies the oral airway, the body reacts as if it is confronting a six-foot tiger threatening its life, setting off a chain reaction throughout the body.

- Low thyroid function—hypothyroidism—is a very common cause of a super-sized tongue. Having hypothyroid properly treated works synergistically with oral appliances to reduce pain, fatigue, and heart disease.

Chapter Seven

A Deeper inside Look
at Sleep Apnea

Ninety-five percent of the Americans with sleep apnea do not know they have sleep apnea and consequently face cardiovascular complications and sudden death.

— William C. Dement, MD[1]

Deep sleep can raise the dead-tired, provided the tongue is not in the airway. The problem: most patients with Impaired Mouth do not know that they sleep with a pinched airway that disrupts their sleep. "Suddenly, I am not half the man I used to be", as the Beatles' song *Yesterday* goes, can simply be a reflection of Impaired Mouth Syndrome.

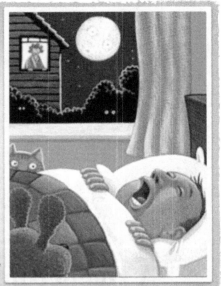

Obstructive Sleep Apnea (OSA) Symptoms:

- High blood pressure, stroke*
- Heart attack, sudden death*
- Diabetes, obesity*
- GERD: acid reflux*
- Lower immunity*
- Depression, anxiety*
- Brain fog, senile memory*
- Accelerated aging*
- Chronic pain*
- Daytime sleepiness, accidents*
- Sleep bruxing (Teeth grinding)

* William C. Dement and Merrill M. Mitler, *JAMA* 269, no. 12 (1993): 1548–1550.

Sleep bruxing in the slide above was not in Dr. Dement's paper, but is added by the author as a proposal.

Obstructive sleep apnea (OSA) is characterized by the collapse of the airway during sleep. Simply, the muscles in the back of the throat relax too much, making normal breathing impossible. The ensuing oxygen deprivation contributes to a long list of mind, body, and mouth symptoms, including teeth grinding and its related complications.

This should be of interest to all patients, health professionals, health insurers, and employers alike because it harms health and raises costs. A 1999 University of Washington study found that medical costs are about two times higher for patients with undiagnosed sleep apnea compared with age- and gender-matched individuals.[2]

In my experience, many dental issues are also the fallout of OSA, including teeth grinding, gum recession, dental sensitivity, bone loss that eventually leads to failed dental work, many root canals, and fractured teeth that require extraction and implants. (Book 2 of the *Holistic Mouth Solutions* series will cover teeth grinding in depth.)

Deadly OSA Is STILL Undetected 75 Percent of the Time

Sleep-disordered breathing (SDB) is the medical term for abnormal breathing patterns during sleep, and it is "associated with considerable morbidity," according to the American Academy of Sleep Medicine. [3] OSA is a common form of SDB.

Daytime sleepiness is a cardinal feature of sleep apnea. Others include waking up tired, jaw clenching, and teeth grinding, which is now called sleep bruxism in sleep medicine.

While 3D-CT imaging can raise clinical suspicion and provide objective evidence, it cannot be used alone to diagnose OSA. Only a doctor trained in sleep medicine can diagnose OSA. An overnight sleep test collects data on brain waves, heart rate, muscle activity (or lack thereof), oxygen levels, and breathing. [4]

A 2002 study in *The Lancet* stated: "OSA can be diagnosed on the basis of characteristic history (snoring, daytime sleepiness) and physical examination (increased neck circumference), but overnight polysomnography [commonly known as a sleep test] is needed to confirm presence of the disorder." [5]

Yet OSA—and SDB in general—still goes largely undiagnosed. The prevalence is high among men and is much higher than previously suspected among women. A 1993 *New England Journal of Medicine* study reported "9 percent of middle-aged women and 24 percent of middle-aged men have undiagnosed SDB." [6]

Fifteen years later, the same researcher found that 75 percent of severe sleep apnea cases had still gone undetected. [7]

How Holistic Mouth Doctors Can Help Screen OSA Cases

The health problems linked with OSA are severe and widespread. Experts estimate that as many as one in four American adults could benefit from a sleep evaluation. I believe every medical and dental patient deserves a screening to rule out airway obstruction as a source of presenting symptoms.

A much overlooked solution is a Holistic Mouth that can support deep sleep and natural recovery. Redeveloping the jaws with the right type of oral appliances can provide just that, bringing the body back to life with a wider airway and deeper sleep.

Given how widespread OSA is—and the prominent role of the mouth in OSA—dentists trained as Holistic Mouth doctors are in a good position to recognize orofacial signs of an impaired mouth and obstructed airway, to screen for OSA (and thereby refer affected patients for sleep tests), and to provide oral-appliance therapy where indicated.

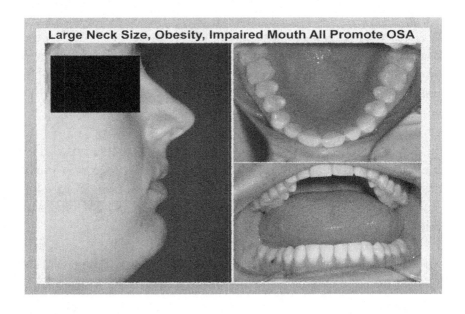

Large Neck Size, Obesity, Impaired Mouth All Promote OSA

A Holistic Mouth checkup can serve as a valuable screening opportunity to catch this costly condition early on. After all, most of the leading causes of OSA start in the mouth, and many signs of "six-foot tiger, three-foot cage" are readily seen during a dental exam:

- A lower jaw that is short compared with the upper jaw (*retrognathia*)

- Certain shapes of the palate or airway that cause the airway to be narrower or collapse more easily

- A large neck—seventeen inches or more in men, sixteen inches or more in women

- A large tongue that can fall back and block the airway

- Obesity

- Large tonsils and adenoids in children that can block the airway[8]

The tongue is the big obstructor in OSA. Freeing the airway of a tongue obstruction using oral appliances as part of an overall wellness program can improve sleep, restore energy, and upgrade life quality for patients, as we shall see in the case studies ahead.

Holistic Mouth Bites

- Snoring, sleep apnea, and teeth grinding all have an impaired mouth as their anatomical source.

- An impaired mouth and pinched airway are the anatomical roots of OSA, with the tongue as the big obstructer. Oxygen deprivation contributes to a long list of mind, body, and mouth symptoms.

- A Holistic Mouth checkup can serve as a valuable screening opportunity to catch this costly condition early on. Dentists trained in Holistic Mouth Solutions can help free the airway of a tongue obstruction to help improve sleep, restore energy, and upgrade life quality for patients.

Chapter Eight

Resolving High Blood Pressure without Medication: Case Study

Half of all OSA patients have high blood pressure.[1] Why? While salt is a well-known culprit, an impaired mouth's contribution to high blood pressure through OSA is virtually unknown. Here is a case of how blood pressure can be lowered when an impaired mouth is treated with oral appliances.

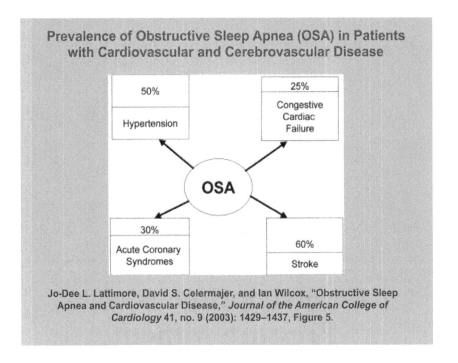

Prevalence of Obstructive Sleep Apnea (OSA) in Patients with Cardiovascular and Cerebrovascular Disease

50%	25%
Hypertension	Congestive Cardiac Failure

OSA

30%	60%
Acute Coronary Syndromes	Stroke

Jo-Dee L. Lattimore, David S. Celermajer, and Ian Wilcox, "Obstructive Sleep Apnea and Cardiovascular Disease," *Journal of the American College of Cardiology* 41, no. 9 (2003): 1429–1437, Figure 5.

B.N. was a forty-six-year-old mom with six kids. She had a family history of heart disease and sought out Holistic Mouth care because:

- She had a medical diagnosis of mild obstructive sleep apnea (OSA). Her sleep test showed an AHI of 11, with very loud snoring 50.2 percent of the time.

- She had woken up tired three to four mornings a week "for as long as I can remember."

- Her medical doctor had recommended continuous positive airway pressure (CPAP), but she had found it impossible to sleep with that mask.

- She had persistent pain across the top of her shoulders and lower back on and off for fifteen years.

- She had high blood pressure and had been on medication for nine years. Her blood pressure was 120/80 mm Hg with medication, and 140/95 without. (Normal is 120/80 more or less, depending on your doctor's belief and criteria.)

Impaired Mouth Clues Uncovered by B.N.'s CSI

Examining B.N.'s teeth and other oral structures, I saw advanced wear and tear on the edges of her upper and lower front teeth, suggestive of teeth grinding—a common finding in patients with a narrowed oral airway. In addition, her upper and lower front teeth were too narrow by 4 mm and 5 mm, respectively, and her uvula was not visible. That, too, is a marker for sleep-apnea risk.

Three-dimensional CT imaging showed she had neck vertebrae misalignment, accounting for her aches and pains, and an airway in the orange-red zone while standing, which means it was more likely to collapse during sleep.

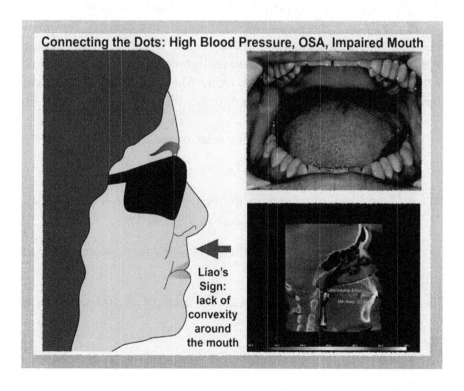

Connecting the Dots: High Blood Pressure, OSA, Impaired Mouth

Liao's Sign: lack of convexity around the mouth

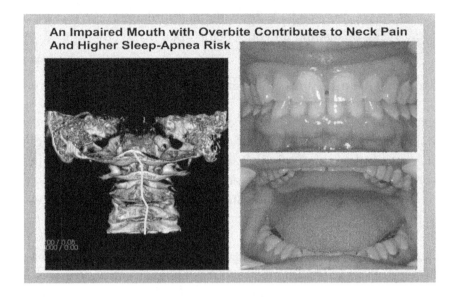

An Impaired Mouth with Overbite Contributes to Neck Pain And Higher Sleep-Apnea Risk

The Holistic Mouth Solutions That B.N. Implemented

B.N. choose oral-appliance therapy over CPAP, so custom oral appliances designed to widen and realign both jaws were made and fitted over her upper and lower teeth. She was instructed to wear them fourteen to sixteen hours a day, including during sleep, and to:

- Turn the gear for widening once a week.

- Return for a progress check once a month.

- Use blackout blinds in the bedroom and no TV, computer screens, tablet, or cell phone in the bedroom.

- Eat a smaller portion of dinner before 7:00 p.m. or four hours before bedtime.

- Have lights out by 10:30, and be asleep by 11:00 p.m. to flow with the circadian rhythm.

Results Produced by Holistic Mouth Solutions for B.N.

After fifteen months of just wearing oral appliances to sleep and without diet and lifestyle changes, B.N. reported that her blood pressure was down by 13/10, from 140/87 to 127/77. Depending on your doctor's criteria, normal blood pressure is either 120/80 millimeter of mercury plus your age, or less than 120/80.[2]

"Now I need to adjust my medication with my doctor," she said. Moreover, she said, "My blood pressure does not shoot up right away like it used to when I forget my medication. My blood pressure now stays normal for a couple of days even when I don't take the meds.

"The aches and pains in my shoulders are improving, too. And I'm not as tired as I used to be—which is important when you're taking care of six kids!"

How can oral-appliance therapy do this? By making the tongue less of an airway obstructor so that her body can sleep in peace, instead of confronting a tiger in her throat.

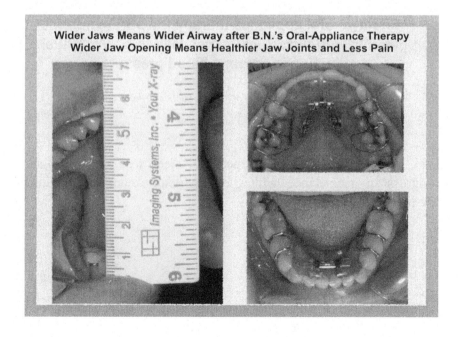

Wider Jaws Means Wider Airway after B.N.'s Oral-Appliance Therapy
Wider Jaw Opening Means Healthier Jaw Joints and Less Pain

According to Japanese research, an individually prescribed oral appliance can lower high blood pressure in patients with mild to moderate OSA by 4.5/3.0 millimeter of mercury over an average of sixty days.[3] B.N.'s drop of 13/10 was much more dramatic, perhaps because she had both upper and lower expander appliances to create a more spacious habitat for her tongue—a point we will return to later.

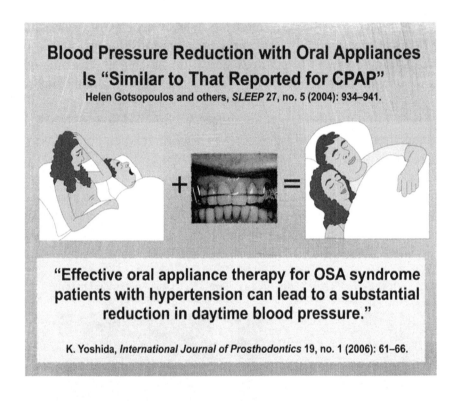

Blood Pressure Reduction with Oral Appliances Is "Similar to That Reported for CPAP"
Helen Gotsopoulos and others, *SLEEP* 27, no. 5 (2004): 934–941.

"Effective oral appliance therapy for OSA syndrome patients with hypertension can lead to a substantial reduction in daytime blood pressure."

K. Yoshida, *International Journal of Prosthodontics* 19, no. 1 (2006): 61–66.

B.N. has been instructed to repeat her sleep test to confirm her progress in accordance with the American Academy of Sleep Medicine guidelines.

Holistic Mouth Bites

- Half of all OSA patients have high blood pressure.

- Blood pressure can be lowered in medically diagnosed OSA patients when an impaired mouth is treated with oral appliances.

- The results can be even more dramatic when both upper and lower appliances are used to create a more spacious habitat for the tongue.

- By considering high blood pressure as a symptom of Impaired Mouth Syndrome, a holistic mouth checkup may help identify pinched airway as a root cause or contributor of sleep apnea and drug-resistant hypertension.

Chapter Nine

Sleep-Apnea Solutions: CPAP Machine Dependence or Oral-Appliance Development?

Oral appliances are indicated for use in patients with mild to moderate OSA who prefer them to continuous positive airway pressure (CPAP) therapy, or who do not respond to, are not appropriate candidates for, or who fail treatment attempts with CPAP.

– American Academy of Sleep Medicine[1]

The results of oral-appliance therapy are predictable when patients follow instructions and recommendations. You are more likely to wake up energized each and every morning if your body can have all the oxygen and sleep it needs.

Many cases of sleep apnea can be treated with oral appliances, but oral appliance therapy is not for every sleep-apnea case. This requires an understanding of OSA case types and treatment guidelines.

Treatment Options for Obstructive Sleep Apnea

Currently, there are four options for treating OSA, according to the American Academy of Sleep Medicine (AASM):

Continuous positive airway pressure (CPAP): CPAP is the standard treatment option for moderate to severe cases of OSA and a good option for mild sleep apnea.

Oral appliances: An oral appliance is an effective treatment option for people with mild to moderate OSA who either prefer it to CPAP or are unable to successfully comply with CPAP therapy. Oral appliances look much like sports mouth guards, and they help maintain an open and unobstructed airway by repositioning or stabilizing the lower jaw, tongue, soft palate, or uvula. They should always be fitted by dentists who are trained in sleep medicine.

Surgery: Surgery is a treatment option for OSA when noninvasive treatments such as CPAP or oral appliances have been unsuccessful. Surgical options may require multiple operations, and positive results may not be permanent.

Behavioral (and sleep-position) changes: Weight loss benefits many people with sleep apnea, and changing from back-sleeping to side-sleeping may help those with mild cases of OSA.[2]

The choice of treatment depends on the severity of the problem per your sleep-test score (AHI) and your personal tolerance and preference. As the 2006 AASM guidelines put it:

> Oral appliances are indicated for use in patients with mild to moderate OSA who meet any of the following criteria:
>
> a) they prefer oral appliances to CPAP therapy;
>
> b) they do not respond to CPAP, are not appropriate candidates for it, or fail treatment attempts with it;
>
> c) they do not respond to, or are not good candidates for, treatment in which behavior is modified, such as losing weight and changing the sleep position.[3]

AASM also recommends that OSA patients should have a follow-up sleep test, that severe OSA patients should start with CPAP because it has been shown to be more effective in severe cases, and that "oral appliances should be fitted by qualified dental personnel who are trained and experienced in the overall care of oral health, the temporomandibular joint (TMJ), dental occlusion, and associated oral structures."

The updated 2015 joint recommendations by AASM and the American Academy of Dental Sleep Medicine (AADSM) emphasized collaboration between sleep medicine doctors and dentists to help patients with snoring and sleep apnea.[4]

Impaired Mouth Syndrome is a set of medical and dental symptoms rooted in deficient jaws and pinched airway. It's helpful to patients if their doctors know the dental symptoms, and their dentists know the medical symptoms of Impaired Mouth Syndrome listed in Holistic Mouth Score.

Holistic Mouth Score

Mouth	Score	Body	Score
Snoring, morning dry mouth	0 1	Gasping or choking in sleep	0 1
Teeth grinding, jaw	0 1	Neck, shoulder, or back pain; headaches	0 1
Mouth breathing, chapped lips	0 1	Erectile dysfunction or PMS	0 1
Persistent/wandering dental sensitivity	0 1	High blood pressure, heart disease	0 1
Gum recession and/or redness	0 1	Diabetes type 2, bloating after meals	0 1
Clicking/locking jaw joints, zigzag jaw opening	0 1	Weight gain, pot belly; acid reflux	0 1
Morning headache and/or sore jaws	0 1	Daytime sleepiness, fatigue	0 1
Deep overbite or underbite (weak chin)	0 1	Senile memory, ADD/ADHD	0 1
Frequent cavities or broken/chipped teeth	0 1	Frequent colds, flu, and skin disorders	0 1
Teeth prints on the sides of the tongue	0 1	Obstructive sleep apnea from a sleep test	0 1
Bony outgrowth on palate or inside lower jaw	0 1	Stuffy/runny nose, scratchy/itchy throat	0 1
Sunken lips and reverse smile curve (sad)	0 1	Forward head: ears ahead of shoulders	0 1
History of teeth extractions for braces	0 1	Waking up to urinate more than once	0 1
Bulge under lower jaw, double chin	0 1	Large neck size (M>17, W>15)	0 1
History of lots of dental work + medical symptoms	0 1	Poor digestion and elimination	0 1
Malocclusion (crowded teeth)	0 1	Depression, anxiety, grouchiness	0 1

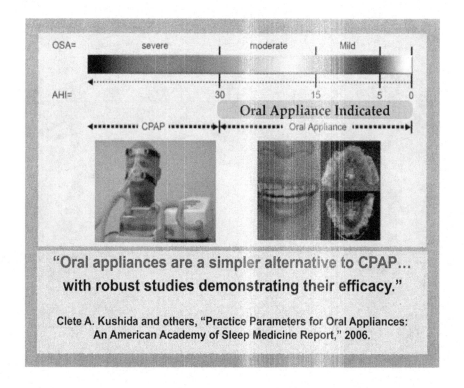

"Oral appliances are a simpler alternative to CPAP... with robust studies demonstrating their efficacy."

Clete A. Kushida and others, "Practice Parameters for Oral Appliances: An American Academy of Sleep Medicine Report," 2006.

CPAP works by using pressurized air to keep the airway from collapsing during sleep, whereas oral appliances work either by holding the lower jaw (and thus the tongue) forward, or by enlarging the "three-foot cage" with oral expander appliances such as B.N.'s.

Oral appliances are "a simpler alternative to CPAP," as a 2010 Canadian Agency for Drugs and Technologies in Health concluded.[5]

"Over the last decade, there has been a significant expansion of the evidence base to support the use of oral appliances, with robust studies demonstrating their efficacy." according to a 2007 Australian study.[6]

In my experience, oral appliances also help to realign skeletal malocclusion and relieve chronic pain in the head, jaws, neck, shoulders, and back.

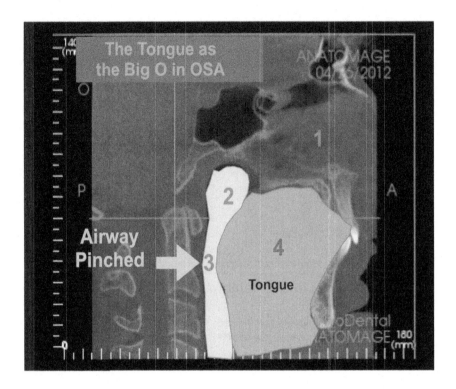

The other key to choosing between CPAP and oral-appliance therapy is patient compliance. After all, the best device or technology in the world is no good if it is not used.

A 1996 Israeli study found that, of the two, oral-appliance therapy was "strongly preferred over the CPAP by the subjects." While both devices significantly decreased the symptoms of excessive daytime sleepiness and were broadly successful, severe cases did do better with CPAP. Yet following up ten months later, the researchers found that nearly all—nineteen of twenty-one—patients continued to use their appliance either nightly or intermittently. Only one was still using CPAP. Only one was using neither.[7]

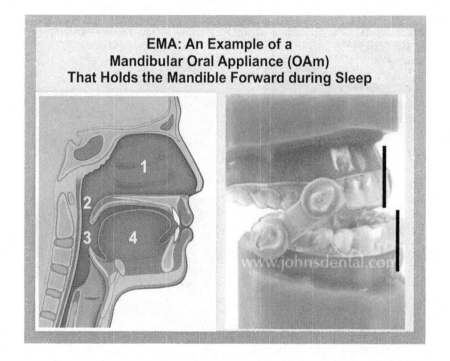

**EMA: An Example of a
Mandibular Oral Appliance (OAm)
That Holds the Mandible Forward during Sleep**

Two Categories of Oral Sleep Appliances

As I write this, there are two categories of oral sleep appliances: one-arch mandibular advancement and biomimetic expanders for 3D widening of upper, lower, or both arches.

Mandibular advancement appliances (MAA or OAm for short) are the more traditional devices. They work by holding the lower jaw in a more forward and open position overnight to keep the tongue out of the throat.

Mandibular Oral Appliance (OAm) Holds Lower Jaw Forward Overnight

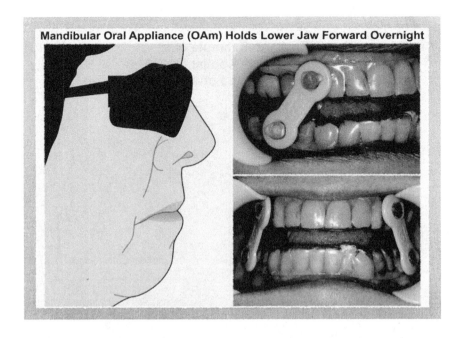

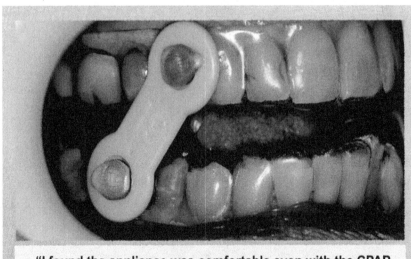

"I found the appliance was comfortable even with the CPAP machine. I also noticed that when breathing my airway seemed bigger, and it was easier to breath even when lying down. Thank you, Dr. Liao."

M.C., Bowie, Maryland

Biomimetic oral appliances (OAb), on the other hand, are similar to retainers or sports mouth guards, with bite alignment and expander features built in. Their actions mimic the 3-D growth of the jaws and the craniofacial skeleton, with a wider airway as a by-product (see chapters 15 and 16).

Both OAm and OAb come in many different designs, each marketed with different claims as to what it can do. What matters to me is not the opinion behind the device but whether it solves the patient's problem at the root so that the body can run itself with greater ease and efficiency. Individual case reports can be useful indicators of treatment merit and clinical experience, especially when supported by science.

For instance, a 1996 study out of Canada found that oral-appliance therapy "is an effective treatment in some patients with mild-moderate OSA and is associated with fewer side effects and greater patient satisfaction than N-CPAP [nasal-CPAP]."[8]

Similarly, a controlled Australian trial by Gotsopoulos afound that over a four-week period, oral-appliance therapy for OSA resulted in "a 50 percent reduction in mean [average] AHI" and "a reduction in blood pressure similar to that reported with CPAP."[9]

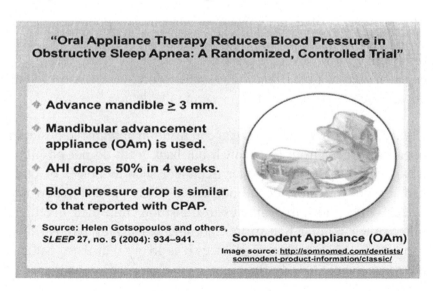

"Oral Appliance Therapy Reduces Blood Pressure in Obstructive Sleep Apnea: A Randomized, Controlled Trial"

- Advance mandible ≥ 3 mm.
- Mandibular advancement appliance (OAm) is used.
- AHI drops 50% in 4 weeks.
- Blood pressure drop is similar to that reported with CPAP.

Source: Helen Gotsopoulos and others, *SLEEP* 27, no. 5 (2004): 934–941.

Somnodent Appliance (OAm)

Image source: http://somnomed.com/dentists/
somnodent-product-information/classic/

"Oral appliances are less efficacious in reducing the AHI," says a 2006 study from University of Western Ontario "but oral appliances appear to be used more (at least by self-report), and in many studies were preferred over CPAP when the treatments were compared." [10]

On the other hand, "CPAP produced the best improvement in terms of physiological, symptomatic, and health-related quality-of-life measures, while the oral appliance was slightly less effective," according to a 2007 study from Hong Kong. [11]

Still, there's a downside to consider with long-term CPAP use: It may cause both jaws to retrude in a direction unfavorable to the airway. This was the finding of a 2010 study: "The use of an nCPAP machine for more than two years may change craniofacial form by reducing maxillary and mandibular prominence and/or by altering the relationship between the dental arches." [12]

As we'll see in more detail shortly, retruded jaws spell bad news for the airway.

The Advantages and Limitations of Mandibular Oral Appliances

The advantage of a mandibular advancement appliance (OAm) is that the therapy is simple and relatively low cost. There are disadvantages however: it does not work in all cases, and it can create jaw-joint (TMJ) and bite issues. Moreover, it is a lifelong dependence—you have to keep wearing the device.

Clinically, long-term use of OAm can result in unintended posterior open bite where front teeth touch but back teeth do not on biting down; that may require further treatment such as braces or other dental work to restore dental occlusion. Many patients report that it takes fifteen to thirty minutes to transition from their overnight bite to their regular bite in the morning when they remove their mandibular advancement appliance. It is likely that these patients have jaw-joint (TMJ) dysfunction.

In my view, posterior open bite is rooted in the unrecognized impaired mouth. Wearing the sleep appliance overnight doubles as a TMJ therapy in these cases; i.e., it's a treatment. So removing it actually reverses the overnight gains. This seesaw effect of OAm does not resolve the cause of their TMJ trouble or sleep apnea, even though it does serve as a useful crutch.

More importantly, both OAm and CPAP manage the airway without answering the question *WHY*: why does the mandible need to be pulled forward, or why is high-pressure air needed to deliver oxygen past choke points in the first place?

"Management" does not mean resolution. After using CPAP or OAm for years, the deficient airway remains. In some cases, this limitation is acceptable, such as for older patients who have mouths full of old dental work that they do not wish to change. The same limitation may not be acceptable to a college student or an adult who prefers to address the root cause once and for all.

In my opinion, leaving out the more important maxilla (upper jaw) amounts to entering the boxing ring with the dominant hand tied behind your back.

The Two-Arch and Superior Alternative: Biomimetic Oral Appliances

Enter biomimetic appliances (OAb), which can actually redevelop a narrow airway from one lane to four. This allows for more oxygen traffic as a by-product of redeveloping jaws orthopedically by restarting your own genetic assembly line to make bone. For this reason, I also refer to them as *epigenetic orthopedic appliances.*

"Biomimetic" means, literally, imitating life. I use biomimetic appliances to turn on craniofacial growth following each adult patient's own genetic blueprint. I can also add features to match each patient's needs: weak chin; snoring; crowded or crooked teeth; bad bite; jaw-joint clicks, pops, or locks; jaw clenching; teeth grinding;

pain or stiffness in and around the mouth; flat midface; and/or thin lips.

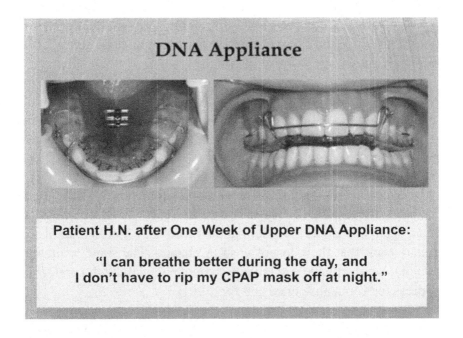

DNA Appliance

Patient H.N. after One Week of Upper DNA Appliance:

"I can breathe better during the day, and I don't have to rip my CPAP mask off at night."

Biomimetic treatment (OAb) is painless because it imitates natural growth during teenage years. OAbs can redevelop the maxilla, the mandible, or both, by:

- Relaxing jaw muscles to reduce or resolve aches and pains naturally

- Aligning jaws orthopedically with the head, neck, and spine

- Increasing jawbone volume so that all crowded teeth fit into the dental arches, with or without braces

- Creating oral volume between the two jaws for the tongue to stay in the mouth and to keep the airway open

- Enlarging the airway in 3-D as a result of redeveloping both jaws and the surrounding craniofacial skeleton

ALF (Advanced Light-wire Functional) is another amazing appliance that targets both the mandible and the more important maxilla, which we will discuss in greater detail in Book 2.

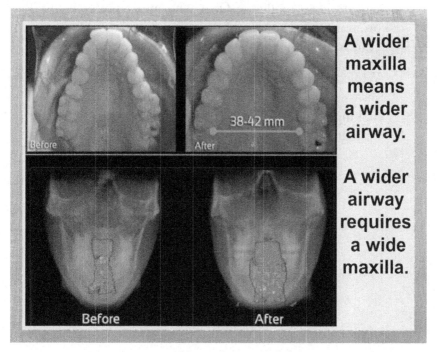

A wider maxilla means a wider airway.

A wider airway requires a wide maxilla.

Images courtesy of Dr. G. Dave Singh

Because mind, body, and mouth are connected, my oral appliance therapy is always part of an overall wellness program to bring the Whole back to higher function and better health.

By targeting the maxilla instead of just the mandible, OAb allows for a fuller expression of genetic potential in the midface and oral airway. This is a game changer as you'll see in the next chapter.

Holistic Mouth Bites

- There are many types of oral appliances. Biomimetic appliances allow us to redevelop the mouth, which in turn widens the airway. They work by signaling stem cells in tooth sockets to make new bone for the jaws.

- An oral appliance is an effective treatment option for people with mild to moderate OSA who either prefer it to CPAP or are unable to successfully comply with CPAP therapy. If your AHI is less than 30, you can use oral appliances.

- While appliances that hold the lower jaw forward have been shown to be helpful for OSA, they cannot come close to making a Holistic Mouth. Biomimetic appliances can by targeting both jaws.

Chapter Ten

The Rarely Addressed Game Changer: The Maxilla

The airway functions, in a real sense, as a keystone for the face.

– Dr. Donald H. Enlow,
Handbook of Facial Growth[1]

The *maxilla*—the medical term for the upper jaw and colored purple in the image below—forms the middle third of the face along with the cheekbones (*zygoma*). The maxilla is a game changer in oral and total health, yet it is rarely addressed in medicine or dentistry.

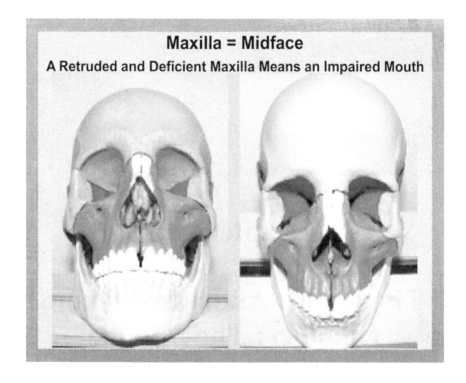

Maxilla = Midface

A Retruded and Deficient Maxilla Means an Impaired Mouth

A well-developed maxilla is a cardinal feature of a Holistic Mouth while a deficient maxilla is the root of an impaired mouth. A fully developed maxilla is a secret to facial attractiveness AND a reliable formula to superior job performance through a wide-open airway and a good night's sleep.

A deficient maxilla is one that's narrow with crowded teeth, shrunken after teeth are pulled and the resulting spaces are closed by braces, retruded (retracted into the head), or some combination of these.

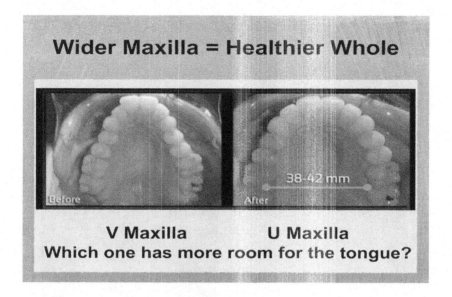

Wider Maxilla = Healthier Whole

V Maxilla   U Maxilla
Which one has more room for the tongue?

The big takeaway: a deficient maxilla is the origin of a narrow airway behind the palate, the tongue, or both. This has life-changing consequences as the case of Chema shows.

The Impaired Mouth that Blocked Conception: The Case of Chema

Before seeking my opinion, Chema, a twenty-eight-year-old software engineer, had gone to the hospital for pain inside her left temple and forehead and in her three upper front teeth that had undergone root canal treatment and were already crowned. After a brain scan and neurological evaluation revealed nothing wrong, the doctors suggested removing the dental work. Chema's main complaints included pain in her upper front teeth and lower left molar, teeth grinding, jaw-joint pain on both sides, and neck and shoulder pain.

Chema turned teary when I asked my usual question: *If your fairy godmother could grant you three wishes regarding your symptoms, what would you wish for?* Her husband had to hold her hand as she told me between sobs about how they had been trying to conceive their first child without success.

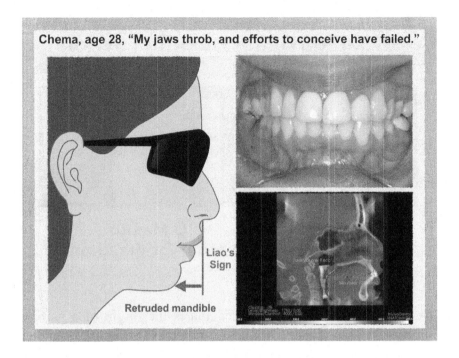

Chema, age 28, "My jaws throb, and efforts to conceive have failed."

Liao's Sign

Retruded mandible

My CSI showed that Chema had been living with undiagnosed Impaired Mouth Syndrome, including a choked airway, weak chin, crowded teeth, tenderness in both jaw joints, and cold hands and feet.

In my view, teeth grinding was the source of pain in her teeth, around her mouth, and inside her head, which stemmed from her pinched airway, which was in the orange-red zone and susceptible to collapse. Her cold hands and feet suggested possible low thyroid function and body temperature. This combination of low thyroid and pinched airway means insufficient energy to support a new life.

I referred Chema for thyroid testing and a sleep test and suggested a diet rich in marine vegetables and minerals and warming spices since she was a very committed vegetarian. She chose oral-appliance therapy and then went to visit her Asian home country soon after starting treatment.

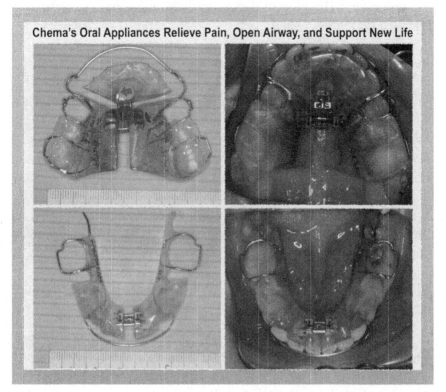

Chema's Oral Appliances Relieve Pain, Open Airway, and Support New Life

Chema's Oral Appliances Relieve Pain, Open Airway, and Support New Life

Chema's Treatment Outcome

"I found out last week that I am six weeks pregnant," Chema told me in an email three and a half months later.

She also reported greatly reduced pain. On a scale of 0 to 10 (none to excruciating pain), Chema reported, "Front teeth pain 3, sleep quality 4, morning energy 3, daytime fatigue 4, teeth grinding 3, and 8 when I forget to wear appliance to sleep."

Whole-body health pays a price when the maxilla is underdeveloped. With two-arch biomimetic oral appliances solving her three-foot-cage problem, Chema was able to support a new life. At six months she reflected, "The biggest difference is no more pain in teeth, and [I] wake up feeling rested."

Recently, she sent me the following:

"I delivered my baby boy 11 months after starting oral appliances. I got really busy after that and so haven't been able to follow up. I have continued to wear the appliance almost every night and I believe it has helped me manage better with the few hours of broken sleep I was getting."

While many factors contribute to difficulties conceiving a baby, an impaired mouth with its pinched airway is a frequently overlooked one.

There is no upside to a deficient maxilla, but there is magic to a fully developed maxilla.

The Secret Source of Radiant Health and an Attractive Face

As documented by Dr. Weston Price, a well-developed maxilla comes with high cheekbones, naturally straight teeth, keen eyesight, a good airway, and facial radiance.[2] Dr. Price's book *Nutrition and Physical Degeneration*—and images like the ones below— catalyzed my turn toward Holistic Mouth Solutions. I keep these images in my mind when I see suffering patients.

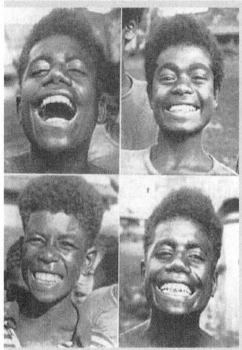

Natural Wellness

Full genetic potential looks like this:

- Broad faces
- Wide arches
- Balanced head and jaws
- High cheekbones
- Radiant energy
- Spontaneous joy
- No need for pediatrician
- No need for braces

Images Courtesy of Sally Fallon, Weston A. Price Foundation.

Facial radiance results from the maxilla doing its job to support alignment, breathing, circulation, digestion, energy, and sleep. In my experience however, a fully developed maxilla is rare among modern Americans.

Indeed, at the end of every CSI into chronic pain and fatigue, there is a maxilla that is either too narrow, retruded, or both. A narrow or retruded maxilla can (and often does) entrap the lower jaw into a retruded position that drives the tongue farther into the throat.

Think of the maxilla as a shoe and the mandible as a foot. The "heel" is left hanging beyond the shoe when the maxilla is underdeveloped. This discrepancy creates a choke zone behind the soft palate and renders the airway susceptible to sleep apnea that is beyond the reach of a mandibular advance appliance (OAm).

Now we can really see how the maxilla is a major player with respect to brain and body alike through sleep and the airway. Anatomically, for instance, the base of the nose is the roof of the mouth, the floor of the eye sockets is the roof of the maxilla, and high cheekbones are connected to a fully developed maxilla.

Developmentally, the jaws and teeth are part of the body's command and control center. That's because they share the same embryological origin as the brain, spinal cord, pituitary gland, and the rest of the nervous system. Structurally, an aligned and balanced craniofacial skeleton means optimal growth, development, and neuro-hormonal functions.

Jaws and Teeth Rank High on the Body's Organizational Chart

Neural tube cells later become:	Neural crest cells later become:
* Brain	* All sensory receptors and
* Central nervous system	proprioceptors
* Spinal cord	* Peripheral nervous system
* Pituitary gland	* Remaining hormonal glands
* Four upper front teeth and the	* Remaining dental system,
bone around them	except enamel

The maxilla and mandible are part of the body's command and control center.

Neurologically, the trigeminal nerve that supplies the maxilla, the mandible, the teeth, the gums, and the jaw muscles is the largest of the twelve cranial nerves covering the head and the gut.

Nutritionally, the maxilla is susceptible to underdevelopment when the diet lacks whole foods and sufficient minerals through the formative years. "There can be no doubt that modern dental-facial problems are encouraged, if not actually caused, by defective diets, by pathological conditions of the nose and throat, and by general poor health," Francis Pottenger, MD, observed in *Pottenger's Cats* [3].

Nutrition by itself, however, will not restore a stunted maxilla in adults. A bone-building diet, such as *Nourishing Traditions Diet* by Sally Fallon[4], is a basic part of a Holistic Mouth treatment plan.

Socially, the maxilla is a major part of "putting your best face forward" and the centerpiece of social identity. A deficient maxilla comes with flat cheekbones and facial profile, and all the disadvantages of an impaired mouth. Conversely, a face with a well-developed maxilla comes with a naturally lovely smile that is pleasing to the eyes.

Take a look at images of movie stars most widely regarded as beautiful or handsome: Julia Roberts, George Clooney, Berenice Bejo, Rock Hudson, and Greta Garbo, for instance. You'll see each has a well-developed midface that is the maxilla.

Diagnostic Clues for Impaired Mouth CSI

Structurally, the maxilla is connected to the central bone in the skull, the *sphenoid* bone, which forms the skull's "hull" with the *occiput* (pillow) bone in the back.

As the "front end" of the craniofacial skeleton, the maxilla can offer valuable diagnostic clues regarding craniofacial misalignment, such as one eye higher, a slanted mouth, a tilted head, or a narrow and asymmetrical palate, such as the case below. Integration of oral-appliance therapy with craniosacral therapy, massage therapy, and chiropractic care is needed in such cases.

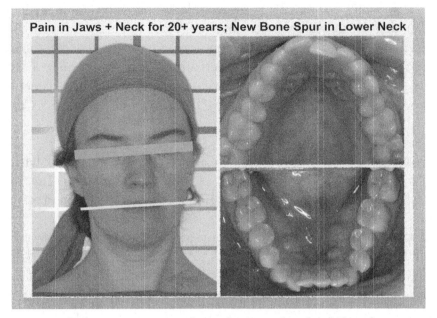

Pain in Jaws + Neck for 20+ years; New Bone Spur in Lower Neck

Red arrow points to neck muscle tension from head tilt and malocclusion. This posture means chronic and persistent pain until the craniofacial imbalance is diagnosed and treated.

Airway: How an Optimal Maxilla Maximizes Academic, Athletic, and Job Performance

Dental-facially, a fully developed maxilla has sufficient arch length and width for all sixteen teeth to line up straight as well as sufficient height to support high cheekbones and big, attractive eyes. Most importantly, a fully developed maxilla comes with a wide-open airway and thus high natural energy from a good night's sleep night after night.

The Teeth Tell the Tale!

STRAIGHT TEETH WIDE Dental Arches	CROOKED, CROWDED TEETH Narrow Dental Arches
Plenty of room in head for pituitary, pineal, hypothalamus	Compromised space for master glands in the head
Good skeletal development, good muscles	Poor development, poor posture, easily injured
Keen eyesight and hearing	Poor eyesight and hearing
Optimal function of all organs	Compromised function of all organs
Optimistic outlook, learns easily	Depression, behavior problems, learning problems
Round pelvic opening, easy childbirth	Oval pelvic opening, difficult childbirth

Slide Courtesy of Sally Fallon, Weston A. Price Foundation

Wide Dental Arches on top left and Narrow Dental Arches on top right added by the author

Watch athletes being interviewed on TV, and you will have opportunities galore to observe the facial features of winners in sports. High cheekbones, wide maxillae, smiles without dark corridors between the teeth and mouth corners, well-defined lower jawlines, and convex facial profiles are the rule—and evidence that Holistic Mouths make winners with optimal form for superior performance.

This isn't to say that someone with an impaired mouth is destined to lose. Sheer will and determination can make winners out of anyone. My point here is that the same athlete, student, or small business owner can perform *better* and achieve *more* while feeling and looking better with a fully developed maxilla as the centerpiece of a Holistic Mouth.

Holistic Mouth Bites

- A deficient maxilla is a cardinal feature of an impaired mouth, and neck pain is a frequent side effect. There is no upside to a deficient maxilla.

- A well-developed maxilla is the foundation of health and beauty, as well as the secret to superior intellectual and athletic performance.

- Pain in and around the head, jaws, neck (and often far beyond) is a frequent finding in patients with Impaired Mouth Syndrome, which happen more frequently in patients who had teeth taken out for braces.

- Developing the maxilla with two-arch biomimetic oral appliances naturally confers a wider airway and more oxygen 24/7. Patients with long-standing pain and other health complaints predictably show rapid improvement once we begin to address the maxilla.

- The same athlete, student, or small business owner can perform *better* and achieve *more* while feeling and looking better with a fully developed maxilla as the centerpiece of a Holistic Mouth.

Chapter Eleven

Holistic Mouth Solutions Ended Fatigue, Allergies, Marital Stress, and Antidepressant Use: Case Study

It is so true that a sleeping issue in a marriage is both parties' problem equally. I am sleeping better because she does not toss and turn OR sound like a walrus.

— K.S.'s spouse

Virtually everything I was trying to fix by removing the mercury had been resolved by opening my airway.

— Patient K.S.

Breathing suffers when the maxilla is structurally deficient. The nasal passage can be regarded as an air tunnel through the maxilla to warm and humidify incoming air and to filter dust, pollen, bacteria, and viruses. Habitual mouth breathing breeds respiratory infections in children and adults alike.

A stuffy nose during developmental years can lead to habitual mouth breathing, narrower jaws, and longer faces, which in turn perpetuate sinus problems in adults. Sinuses are hollow functional spaces inside the maxilla to reduce the weight of the head and to make nitric oxide, which can help relax blood vessels and reduce blood pressure.

A wider maxilla improves nasal breathing. You can experience the difference for yourself right now: Gently seal your lips and exhale normally through your nose. Then place the index fingers of both hands on either side of your nose at nostril level and lightly spread the skin sideways toward your ears. Now inhale through your nose and note the air volume passing through. Most people can feel the difference right away.

Mandibular advancement appliances (OAm) for snoring and sleep apnea cannot help the nasal passage, whereas a biomimetic appliance (OAb) for the maxilla can, naturally and in a lasting way, as we shall see next.

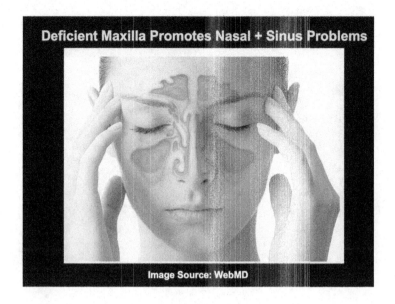

Deficient Maxilla Promotes Nasal + Sinus Problems

Image Source: WebMD

A Solution to Sinus Symptoms in a Dental Office? Yes!

K.S., a thirty-nine-year-old hair stylist, initially came to me about getting her amalgams replaced. "I want to clean up my body because I've been rough on my health for many years."

She described occupational exposure to chemicals and low back pain from a car accident and kickboxing. "At one point, I couldn't work for two months," she said. "I lost my memory while I had a metallic taste in my mouth due to fatigue. I was smoking until last year, and I was on antidepressants for seven years. Then I went vegan one and a half years ago and feel much better. Now I have a bad tooth, and my husband complained about my bad breath."

She also complained of a potbelly she could never seem to lose, despite plenty of exercise and a conscientious diet.

But there was one thing K.S. didn't mention: her sinus issues. But why should she? She did not expect to find a solution to them in a dental office. She did not know about impaired mouth and its connection to the upper airway.

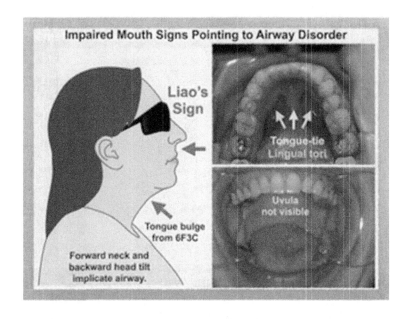

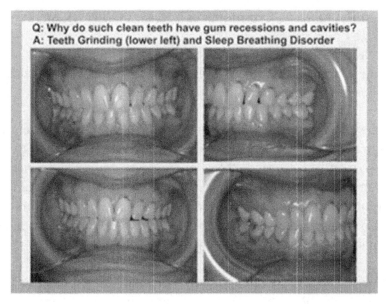

My Holistic Mouth checkup for K.S. revealed the following:

- Her uvula was not visible, indicating a high risk for obstructive sleep apnea (OSA) (more on that in chapter 13).

- Her upper jaw was retruded by 17 mm and was narrower than her lower jaw by 8 mm; this will seriously squeeze her tongue's habitat and crowd her airway.

- There was evidence of teeth grinding with matching wear facets and generalized gum recession

- She had tongue-tie (yellow arrows) and bony overgrowths inside her mandible (green arrows), which are caused by jaw clenching and teeth grinding.

- She had reduced maximal jaw opening of 43 mm between the upper and lower front teeth. (A normal maximal jaw opening is 48 to 52 mm.)

- She had an abscessed tooth, which was the source of her bad breath and which she chose to have extracted.

K.S. chose not have a sleep test done, as recommended, because her insurance deductible was about the cost of her oral-appliance therapy.

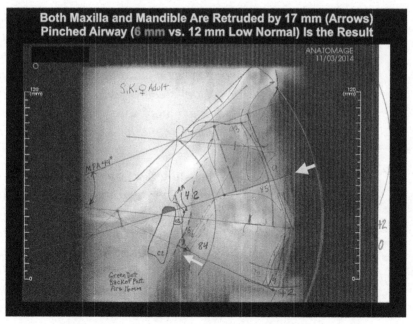

*The yellow arrows point to substantial retrusion of both
the maxilla and mandible pinching the airway.*

K.S.'s Holistic Mouth Solutions Treatment Plan

Starting treatment, K.S. was instructed to wear her custom oral appliances, upper and lower, for sixteen hours a day, expanding them by a quarter of a millimeter each week. During sleep, she was to wear an oral face mask to help nudge her retruded maxilla in the right direction.

She was also given diet and sleep hygiene instructions, orofacial myofunctional therapy to break her habit of mouth breathing, and breathing exercises to unblock her stuffy nose as needed. Holistic Mouth Solutions emphasizes nasal breathing 24/7 to augment maxilla redevelopment. Once a month, she would come into the office for progress checks.

Only Three Months Later ...

After three months, K.S. emailed me:

> *First and foremost, I am experiencing much better sleep, and I am actually dreaming vividly almost every night now! This began happening during the FIRST WEEK of use! I used to have dreams like this when I was a kid, but before using this appliance, not in YEARS! I am sleeping all the way through the night as well. I am so much more awake and alert in the mornings, and all the way throughout the day, for that matter.*
>
> *As for the side effects, I am seeing my skin glowing, my eyes are brighter, and the bags under my eyes are gone! I feel like my circulation all around is much better, and I do not "gasp" for air anymore. Before, I would take [various brand-named allergy medications], nasal spray and gels, humidifiers, tea kettles, exotic muds and salves—you name it! Nothing would prevent me from going to bed fine and waking up stuffed up like hell and feeling like I was going to suffocate! Oh, and that is during NON-allergy season.*

During allergy season (or a bad allergy day), I would just be stuffed up constantly and medicate myself to the point of exhaustion. Now, I take nothing. I now sleep all the way through the night, and I wake up renewed and refreshed.

I was skeptical trying this out. I had braces in the past and did not offer any resistance to the plan to remove two of my front teeth and "shrink" my upper jaw, effectively shrinking the "tiger's cage" too small to allow normal growth or function. When seeing Dr. Liao, he saw this right away and recommended strongly that I be tested for a narrowed airway. I did not come for this: I came to have mercury amalgam fillings removed, so I was unsure. Dr. Liao took the time to explain to me that, despite my legitimate concern about the fillings, my priority should be to open the airway that had become so narrow that it, unbeknownst to me, affected almost every area of my life.

... I opted to have both upper and lower appliances made to increase the size of my jaws, and braces and two false teeth installed later on to hold the shape of my new bite pattern.

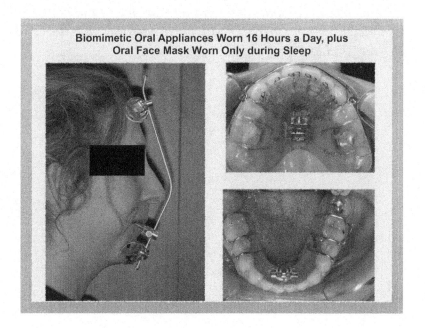

Biomimetic Oral Appliances Worn 16 Hours a Day, plus Oral Face Mask Worn Only during Sleep

This was to take place over the course of two to three years' time, and was to cost a significant amount of money.

The appliance(s) began to work immediately, and since they are to be adjusted weekly (easily by us right at home with a small tool provided), they continue to open the airway more and more every day, allowing me to experience these results to an even greater degree as I go.

I even had a flight recently to California (from Virginia), and I had NO ear pain or discomfort! I used to have to take a bunch of pills and wear [earplugs for airplane travel], and it would STILL kill my ears to fly, but not now.

I never knew that I was being deprived of the oxygen I needed to thrive, but now that I am experiencing it for the first time in my adult life, I regret not looking into having this done YEARS ago!

I highly recommend this to anyone who feels stuffed up in the morning, tired and groggy all day, or any of the plethora of other symptoms associated with a narrowed airway. Thank you, Dr. Liao!

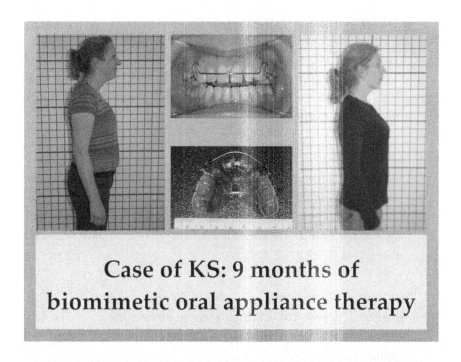

Case of KS: 9 months of biomimetic oral appliance therapy

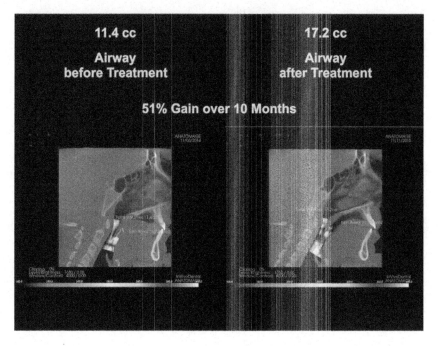

K.S.'s husband added his observations:

I concur from what I have witnessed (which is pretty much everything except the flight). She sleeps better and QUIETER! ... She sleeps in the same spot, and I am now able to get through the night without waking up.

She also clearly has more energy. She thinks better, too, and remembers things that she used to forget. Overall, she just seems more alert and aware that she is alive. She also looks better, too. Her skin looks nice, and her eyes look whiter. I am so impressed that she has had such great results in such a short time.

To those considering, this WILL work if you stick to the program! It may just change your partner's life, too! We both hope that you share this with anyone it can help. Thank you again!

Holistic Mouth Bites

- Eating well, exercising, detoxifying, and other aspects of "living clean" can only help so much if the airway is still too narrow from maxilla deficiency.

- Impaired Mouth Syndrome is an apt diagnosis for KS, since her medical and dental symptoms are resolved when her impaired mouth structure is redeveloped.

- Redeveloping the maxilla helps the sleep partner as well as the sufferer of the impaired mouth and pinched airway.

- Widening the airway can bring relief from chronic stuffiness and allergies, as well as fatigue and being persistently overweight.

Chapter Twelve

The Maxilla Triple Win: Better Sleep, Better Health, Better Looks

A doctor's primary responsibility is to put patients in a position to heal themselves.

— Terrence O'Shaughnessy, DMD, Orthodontist and TMJ Expert

Deficient maxilla development is a hugely overlooked cause of teeth crowding, sinus problems, snoring, sleep apnea, teeth grinding, pain, and fatigue. Development is the change in size, content, and form over time. Many medical, dental, and mood symptoms in adults are downstream consequences of impaired genetic expression during the childhood years.

The maxilla's development is particularly susceptible to epigenetic interferences, starting with tongue-tie at birth that hinders breast-feeding and continuing with pacifiers, nutritional imbalance from manufactured foods after weaning, and the resulting stuffy nose and tonsillar inflammation.

Left uncorrected, nasal obstruction can lead to habitual mouth breathing, initiating a chain reaction that culminates in an impaired mouth and its associated oral-systemic complications.

Tongue-tie (medically called short lingual frenulum) "may lead to abnormal orofacial growth early in life, a risk factor for development of Sleep Disordered Breathing."[1]

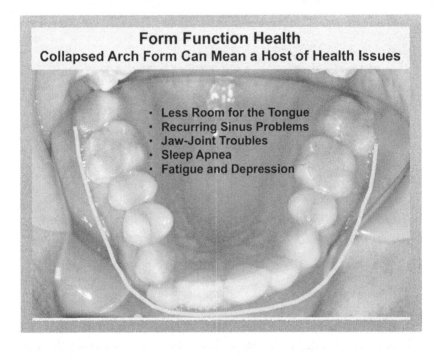

In the image above, you can see a maxilla with significant crowding. In the image below, you can see Liao's Sign indicating the same maxilla as being retruded. This combination results in a weak chin. The deep chin groove signals a low ceiling in the three-foot den, and a big double chin represents the tongue bursting beyond its habitat.

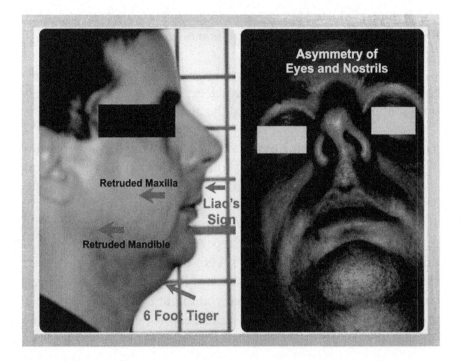

In this severe case, oral-appliance therapy worked as an assist to his CPAP device. His oxygen debt was so huge that it's taken him five years to begin feeling better.

Want to Lose a Weak Chin or Double Chin? Mind Your Maxilla!

A double chin can result from obesity or from the tongue bulging beyond its confines inside a three-foot cage—or both. Normally, the mandible should fit into the maxilla like a foot into a shoe. A deficient maxilla starts a domino effect impacting the airway, facial appearance, and the whole body, often in combination with a retruded mandible..

A retruded maxilla shows up as a flat or a sunken midface in appearance, raising the risk of a retruded mandible and perpetuating snoring and OSA. It is also much harder to treat, with jaw surgery being an option in severe cases. That is why I recommend that children be evaluated by age eight to catch a retruded maxilla while the craniofacial skeleton is still quite malleable.

The height and depth of the orofacial region is assessed from the side. Is the profile protruded or retruded? Does the face round outward, or does it appear pulled back toward the airway?

Treatment for retrusion is *protraction*, or drawing the jaw forward. Protraction is done with either surgery or an oral face mask worn with oral appliances during sleep.

Jaw surgery (*maxillo-mandibular advancement*) to advance the maxilla and mandible has been reported as an effective option to treat OSA.[2] It can be useful in severe cases of obesity and severe skeletal malocclusion. Yet 99 percent of the time, the oral face mask works very well. Contrary to what you might think at first glance of the device, 90 percent of patients can sleep with the oral face mask without any problem.

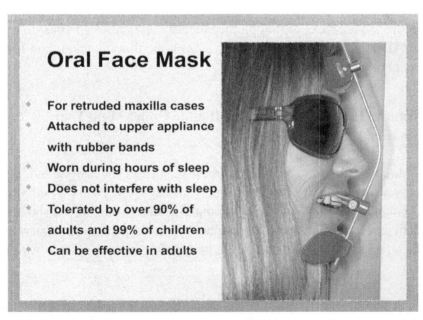

Oral Face Mask

* For retruded maxilla cases
* Attached to upper appliance with rubber bands
* Worn during hours of sleep
* Does not interfere with sleep
* Tolerated by over 90% of adults and 99% of children
* Can be effective in adults

A pair of rubber bands connect the upper oral appliance to the oral face mask.

How a Marvelous Maxilla Is a Missing Key to Optimal Health

49 percent of upper jaws are retruded, based on a study on children by Dr. James McNamara.[3] This is the start of a narrow airway behind the soft palate or tongue, ie, impaired mouth and pinched airway.

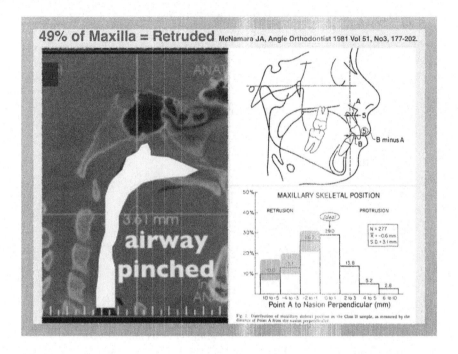

Unrecognized and untreated, children with retruded maxillae may well grow into adults with sleep apnea and all its medical, dental, and mental side effects. This may explain the prevalence of sleep apnea at a later age.

In adults, retruded maxilla is the structural source of a variety of physical features and unfavorable adaptations, including:

○ The white part of the eyes visible between the lower eyelids and the iris[4]

○ The outer corners of the eyes angling downward[5]

- ○ Flat cheekbones and receded midface

- ○ An excessively prominent or deviated nose

- ○ A flat or sunken upper lip in profile (Liao's Sign)

- ○ A narrow and steep palate with little room for the tongue

- ○ Crowded lower and/or upper front teeth

- ○ Clicking, popping, or locking jaw joints (TMJ dysfunction)

- ○ Wrinkles around lips, saggy mouth, and deep facial creases

- ○ A weak chin and/or a double chin or bulge in front of the neck

- ○ A narrow airway

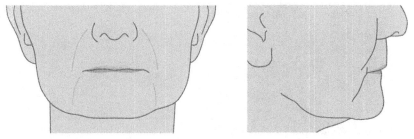

This retiree has fatigue, history of many crowns and root canals, declining memory, and back pain. She also has a deficient airway.

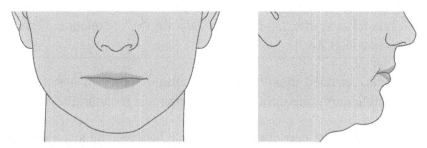

This college girl and a soccer player is heading toward the same medical-dental fate as the librarian.

Redeveloping Retruded Maxilla in Adults

A non-surgical treatment for a retruded maxilla is an oral face mask (OFM) worn during the hours of sleep. Imagine have your maxilla heading in the right direction while you sleep -- what can be better?!

A pair of rubber bands connect the OFM to a maxillary (upper) oral appliance provide a light forward stretch. This light stretch simulates a retruded maxilla to grow in the right direction to open up the airway.

Contrary the first glance, an oral face mask mask is easy to use, and predictably effective. Over 90% patients can sleep with it after a brief period of adjustment. Oral face mask shown below has been used in growing children for decades.[6] It's almost never used in adults until now.

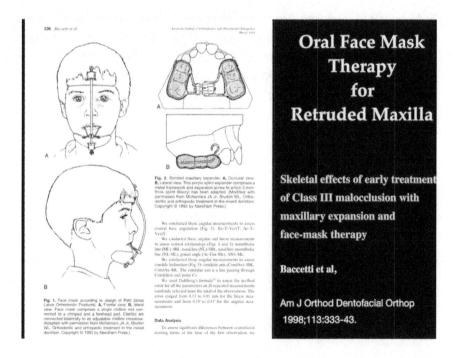

To confirm diagnosis of a retruded maxilla, mandible, or both, I use cephalometric analysis to show me what's off with the "three-foot

cage", where, and by how much. *Cephalometry* is the geometric measurement of the teeth and jaws inside the craniofacial skeleton. It's like an architect's blueprint of the house of the jaws, teeth, and tongue that also tells me if oral face mask is needed in each case.

I have used oral face mask routinely with upper jaw appliance in adults with good results in compliant patients. "Your compliance drives your treatment success" is my advice.

Evidence of Oral Face Mask's Value

S.A., a very motivated CEO in his fifties, wore his oral face mask religiously for two years and gained 10 mm of height in his former three-foot cage. "Every millimeter I gain is a plus for my health," S.A. said. "So why not get the most out of my treatment?!"

S.A.'s airway volume grew by 58 percent from faithfully wearing an oral face mask during sleep and oral appliance twelve to fifteen hours a day over two years. Cephalometrics show that OFM did reduce his maxilla retrusion by 10 mm over 2 years. Look for the change in the size of the yellow dot in the next two slides.

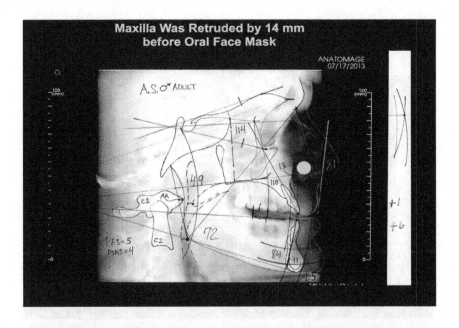

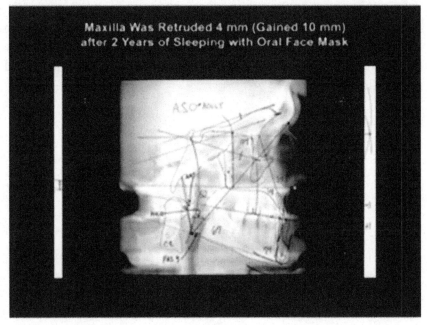

This evidence shows that "the earth is no longer flat" — that the maxilla can indeed be redeveloped and repositioned in 57 year-old with a seriously retruded maxilla.

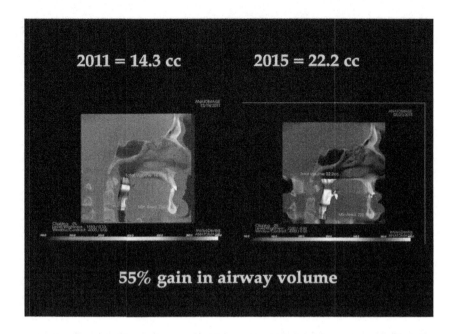

The more retruded the maxilla, the more likely the airway obstruction behind the palate. The more retruded the maxilla, the more likely the mandible is retruded, and this has both medical and dental implications.

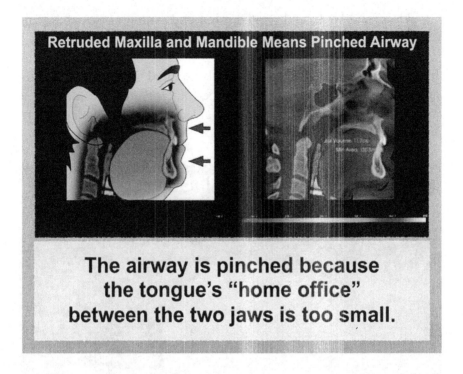

Retruded Maxilla and Mandible Means Pinched Airway

The airway is pinched because the tongue's "home office" between the two jaws is too small.

The more retruded the mandible is, and the more likely we will find the tongue clogging the airway. This can lead to snoring and a higher risk of sleep apnea with its many associated cardiovascular, cancer, and Alzheimer's brain consequences. A 2008 Japanese study made a significant link between a retruded mandible and obstructive sleep apnea.[8]

Airway can be improved predictably, sleep can deepen naturally, and the body restarts with vigor, when a retruded maxilla is recognized and treated, as the case of S.A. shows.

Retruded Jaws: The Real Causes of TMJ Dysfunction that Almost No One Treats

Retruded maxilla and/or mandible come(s) with dental and TMJ (clicking, popping, locking jaw joints) troubles. TMJ Dysfunction (TMJD) is a syndrome covering the pains in the head, neck, face, shoulders, and back, and related mind-body-mouth distress is well documented.[7]

In my experience, TMJD is easily treated by identifying its anatomical source: an underdeveloped and/or retruded maxilla, a retruded mandible, or both. This has an added benefit: wider airway for superior sleep and natural health.

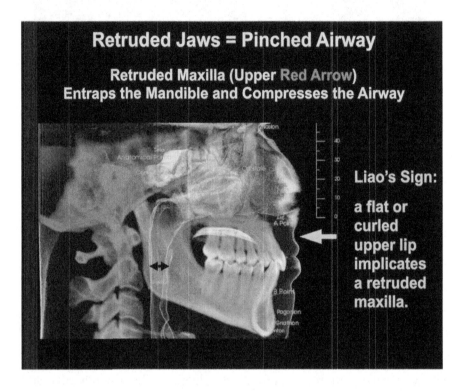

The mandible can even become entrapped—locked into a retruded position — by a deep overbite. With mandibular entrapment comes persistent aches and pains, fatigue, the global symptoms of TMJD, and major complications from teeth grinding, such as broken teeth, loosened dental work, and failed implants, and more.

Beside genetics, a retruded mandible has three developmental (epigenetic) causes:

1. An underdeveloped maxilla with crowded teeth and a narrow arch

2. A retruded maxilla resulting in a narrower airway behind the soft palate

3. A deep overbite, with the upper front teeth inclined toward the palate

Pinkie Test for TMJ and Mandibular Entrapment

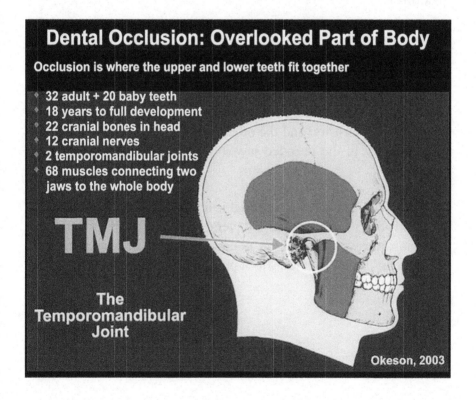

To see if your TMJ/mandible is retruded, you can do a "pinkie" test.

Put your small fingers inside your ear openings with the finger pads facing forward. Feel for the jaw joints pushing against your finger pads when you bite your teeth together, and listen for clicking, popping, or grating sounds. Such sounds suggest entrapment of the lower jaw and a tongue that is pinching the airway.

Next, repeat the same pinkie test, only bite your front teeth together instead. This simulates the protruded position of the jaw joints. If the clicking noise and the pushback go away, then one or both jaws may be retruded.

How to Reach Your Genetic Potential by Freeing Your Trapped Mandible

Freeing the mandible from its entrapment can be an effective way to redevelop the airway naturally and actualize genetic potential.

Lower jaw posture can influence gene expression. In a 2003 study, Dr. Fuentes measured gene activities in rats with one jaw joint induced into retrusion and the other into protrusion. She found less gene activity in the retruded jaw joint and more in the protruded joint.[9]

This means fuller genetic potential is actualized when the mandible is freed from entrapment. Conversely, living with mandibular retrusion means not reaching genetic potential in form, function, health, and life. This study was a huge inspiration to me.

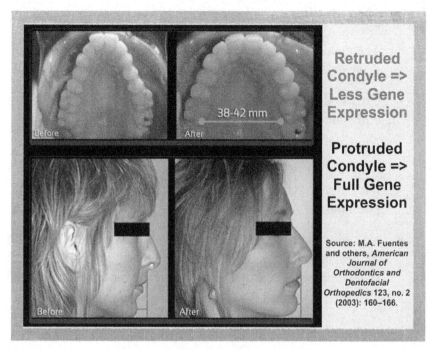

Retruded Condyle => Less Gene Expression

Protruded Condyle => Full Gene Expression

38-42 mm

Before

After

Before

After

Source: M.A. Fuentes and others, *American Journal of Orthodontics and Dentofacial Orthopedics* 123, no. 2 (2003): 160–166.

Images courtesy of Dr. G. Dave Singh

Conclusion: The body can better heal itself when the jaws are positioned so the mandible is freed from entrapment, which in turn requires a fully developed maxilla.

Are your lower front teeth crowded? Going back to the maxilla as the shoe and the mandible as the foot analogy, that means your maxilla is underdeveloped in the "toe box," or retruded in position.

Other surface signs of maxilla deficiency can include a weak chin, a deep chin cleft, double chin, abnormal head posture, and Liao's Sign: a flat or curled upper lip in profile.

Holistic Mouth Bites

- The maxilla is the centerpiece of the face and its development drives mandibular and airway development, or lack thereof.

- Crowded lower front teeth is a clue that the upper jaw's front end is underdeveloped.

- Fuller genetic potential is better actualized when the mandible is freed from entrapment. Conversely, living with mandibular retrusion means a life of not reaching genetic potential.

- Retruded maxilla can be treated in adults with a combination of oral appliances, and oral face mask appears to boost redevelopment in adults with impaired mouth and pinched airway.

Chapter Thirteen

The Telltale Tongue

There are no specific diseases; there are only specific-disease conditions.

– Florence Nightingale (attributed)

The tongue is a big, powerful, muscular organ inside the head, yet it has not received the attention it deserves. Its size, position, and habit matter greatly to maxilla development, orthodontic success, total health through airway and sleep, or initiating Impaired Mouth Syndrome.

Although the tongue is attached to the lower jaw, its parking spot is on the palate where it serves as a natural palate expander in children, doubling in size from birth to adulthood when it serves as a natural palatal retainer. During that time, oral-facial development can (and often does) go wrong, resulting in a three-foot cage.

Another prerequisite for a fully developed maxilla is the absence of a tongue-tie—an abnormal attachment of the tongue to the mandible that prevents full range of motion and agility. Medically, it's known as a *short lingual frenulum*, and you might be surprised by its influence on total health.

Soft Tissues Shape the Skeleton and Your Face Is No Exception

Genetically, humans are coded for a wide-open airway inside a fully developed cranial skeleton with a full face on the outside and room inside for all thirty-two permanent teeth – yes, wisdom teeth included.

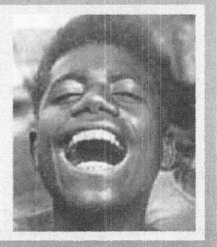

Full Genetic Potential in the Craniofacial Region

* Sufficient maxilla and mandible bone volume for all 32 teeth

* Optimal airway results from fully developed craniofacial skeleton

* Prerequisite: available stem cells, regardless of age

* Stem cells are in sutures around the maxilla and inside tooth sockets of both jaws

In craniofacial growth and development, it is the soft tissues that shape the bones. "According to Moss, the form of the facial skeleton is largely secondary and adaptive to surrounding soft tissues and functional spaces", writes Dr. G.D. Singh in *Epigenetic Orthodontics in Adults*,[1]

Translated: the tongue helps grow its habitat space through normal functions such as suckling, swallowing in the first few months, and chewing and speaking after teeth come in. In the first months of life, the tongue milks the breast by trapping the nipple against the palate. This action is a powerful stimulus to develop the maxilla and craniofacial skeleton through the sutures that join all the skull bones into a head.

Tongue-tie can block this natural, gene-directed development as can habitual mouth breathing. Remember: The tongue participates in the vital function of swallowing 1,000 to 1,500 times a day, every day. This powerful, repetitive pattern can even undo daily chiropractic adjustments or oral-appliance work!

Underdevelopment (an impaired mouth and pinched airway) happens when growth is turned off prematurely by epigenetic factors. The genes are not fully expressed, and the jaw structures do not reach full potential.

In my mind, craniofacial redevelopment reaches full genetic potential when the lower front teeth are no longer crowded and the entire lower arch can fit into the arch peak-to-valley without jaw-joint clicking, popping, and deviations, and enough oral volume for the tongue to stay out of the airway 24/7.

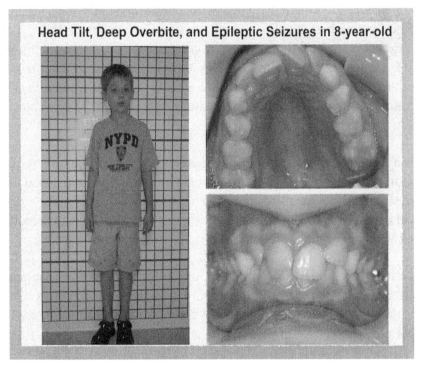

Head Tilt, Deep Overbite, and Epileptic Seizures in 8-year-old

Bad posture and bad bite inside impaired mouth
may be connected -- see chapter 17

Childhood Origins of Impaired Mouth and How to Prevent Needless Suffering

Evidence that the tongue is a big player in OSA comes in part from research in pediatric sleep apnea. A 2015 study from Taiwan concluded that a short lingual frenulum (tongue-tie) "may lead to abnormal orofacial growth early in life, a risk factor for development of SDB [Sleep Disordered Breathing]."[2]

Soft-Tissue Functions Provide the Forces That Shape the Jaws and Bite

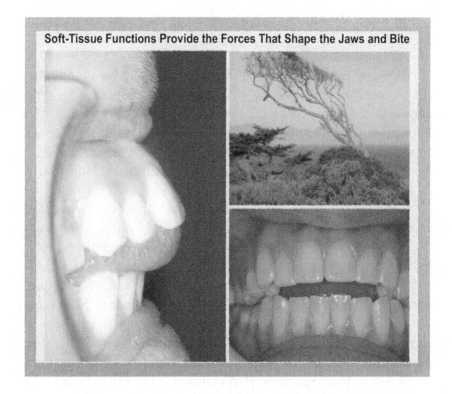

Correct muscle functions in chewing, breathing, swallowing, and mandibular rest posture favor the development of a Holistic Mouth. For example, the lips should be gently sealed and the jaws relaxed when the mouth is at rest and when sleeping.

Abnormal oral-facial muscle use, on the other hand, perpetuates muscle tension and promotes relapse after orthodontics. Swallowing should not be accompanied by a gurgling sound, tension lines around the mouth, or head-bobbing. That's why treatment with Holistic Mouth Solutions includes more than just oral-appliance therapy—and why orofacial myofunctional therapy is important when indicated.

Oral-Facial Myofunctional

Myofunctional therapy is physical therapy for the tongue and all the orofacial muscles involved in swallowing and breathing. (*Myo* comes from the Greek word for *muscle*.) For this reason, it's also known as orofacial myofunctional therapy (OMT). According to the Academy of Applied Myofunctional Sciences, OMT is done through "neurological re-education exercises to assist the normalization of the developing or developed craniofacial structures and function."[3]

Dr. Christian Guilleminault, considered the father of pediatric sleep apnea, did a follow-up study on twenty-four children previously diagnosed with sleep-disordered breathing at ages three and a half to seven years and appropriately treated with tonsillectomy and orthodontics. Thirteen of the twenty-four did not complete myofunctional therapy. All thirteen had a recurrence of SDB (sleep disordered breathing) and mouth breathing during sleep while the eleven who completed myofunctional therapy did not. "This study illustrates the potential importance of myofunctional treatment as an adjunctive treatment [for children with SDB]," wrote Dr. Guilleminault.[4]

Why is myofunctional therapy needed in the first place? Tongue-tie, in varying degrees, is one big reason that is frequently overlooked in childhood.

Tongue-Tie: Baby Lucy's Story

The tongue is a muscular organ capable of movement in all directions. A tongue-tie, or *ankyloglossia*, restricts the tongue to the floor of the mouth by a ligament called a *lingual frenum* (also called *frenulum*). The length and flexibility of a tongue's frenum determines its resting posture.

Imagine the tongue on a short, stiff leash, preventing it from reaching the palate. This is what tongue-tie does. It can lead to excessive chin, as in the facial profile of a witch. Combined with habitual mouth breathing, it can lead to a long, narrow, "horsey" face with a pinched airway inside.

Tongue-tie effectively anchors the tongue to the floor of the mouth and keeps it from reaching the palate where it naturally stimulates maxilla development. A tongue-tie makes it hard for a baby to latch, leading to one frustrated baby and one exhausted new mom. Sixty-nine percent of lactation consultants believe tongue-tie in a newborn can interfere with breast-feeding.[5]

A severe tongue-tie can result in breast-feeding unless the tongue-tie is surgically released (revised). Here's an email I received from a patient and mom to new baby Lucy:

> *We proceeded with the tongue-tie and lip-tie revision, as you had recommended. Lucy is recovering well, and I could tell an immediate difference in her latch. She's still relearning how to use her tongue well, but I'm hopeful this will have a positive impact on her breast-feeding and her oral development. The whole family will see you soon.*

At her last checkup and cleaning, Mom reported that Lucy had more than caught up with her weight.

Poor latch is one sign of tongue-tie, and feeding fatigue is another. Educating new moms about tongue-tie is important. Lucy is lucky to have had her tongue-tie diagnosed in the first few weeks of life. A new protocol was introduced in 2012 to evaluate tongue-tie in newborns relative to feeding fatigue, which is characterized by less than one hour between feedings, fewer sucks, and longer pauses between groups of sucking.[6]

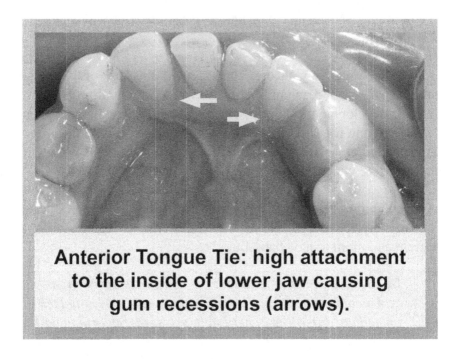

Anterior Tongue Tie: high attachment to the inside of lower jaw causing gum recessions (arrows).

Tongue-Tie Initiates Impaired Mouth

Adults suffering from an impaired mouth's many oral-systemic symptoms often grew up with unrecognized tongue-tie, as well as things like bottle-feeding, pacifiers, poor dietary habits, stuffy nose, and habitual mouth breathing in their childhood. They simply did not have the benefit of a Holistic Mouth checkup while they were growing up.

Even mild to moderate tongue-tie can have dental consequences and subsequent snoring and sleep apnea. Varying degrees of tongue-tie are common among patients who come to see me for teeth grinding and related oral-systemic problems. This is the long shadow of unrecognized tongue-tie from childhood.

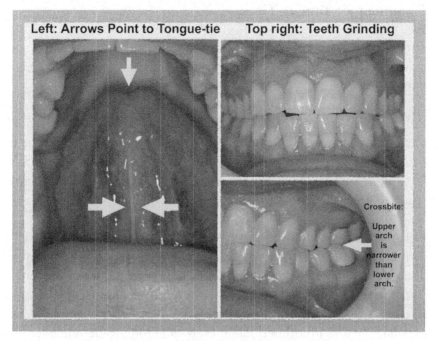

*Here, moderate tongue-tie results in mild crossbite in
the molars and severe fatigue from sleep apnea.*

According to a 2015 Taiwan study, "Children with untreated short frenulum [frenum] developed abnormal tongue function early in life with secondary impact on orofacial growth and SDB [sleep-disordered breathing]."[7] The authors concluded that tongue-tie may "lead to abnormal orofacial growth early in life, a risk factor for development of SDB [sleep-disordered breathing]. Careful surveillance for abnormal breathing during sleep should occur in the presence of short lingual frenulum."

Dental offices trained to provide Holistic Mouth checkups are a good place to monitor tongue-tie and orofacial development.

Treatment for Tongue-Tie

Tongue-tie is treated with a combination of surgical release and myofunctional therapy to free the tongue and oral-appliance therapy to make room for it.

Release of a tongue-tie does not mean cutting or clipping. "To cut" means to detach, while "to release" means to *liberate*. The tongue is *freed* with a surgical release called *lingual frenectomy*, after which the tongue will suddenly have a much wider reach while still being attached.

Releasing tongue-tie is a simple procedure that can be done at birth in a hospital without anesthesia. In older children, frenectomy is done in a dental office using laser and topical numbing gel only. There is little or no pain, and recovery takes less than a day or two. In cases of very narrow jaws, it may be necessary to use a palatal expander before myofunctional therapy and tongue-tie release.

Equally important as the surgical release is the orofacial myofunctional therapy, starting that same day. Properly practiced until correct swallowing is automatic, it can develop or redevelop the tongue's tone and posture. According to the Academy of Orofacial Myofunctional Therapy, a wide variety of other benefits have been reported, including:

- Airway development

- Normalizing oral functions and mitigating sleep disorders [8]

- Correcting oral dysfunction in chewing, swallowing, and speaking

- Stretching tethered oral tissues (tongue- and lip-ties)

- Remedying TMJ disorder

- Guiding healthy craniofacial development

- Relieving orofacial pain

- Helping orthodontic results hold, minimizing relapse

- Providing early intervention to avoid developmental consequences

- Improving brain function and neuroplasticity

- Healing chronic pain with myofunctional connections[9]

The two cases below show just how powerful orofacial myofunctional therapy can be. Orthodontics was stopped and an oral face mask was used in the first case while the second simply closed her lips during the day and slept with her oral face mask attached to her maxillary appliance.

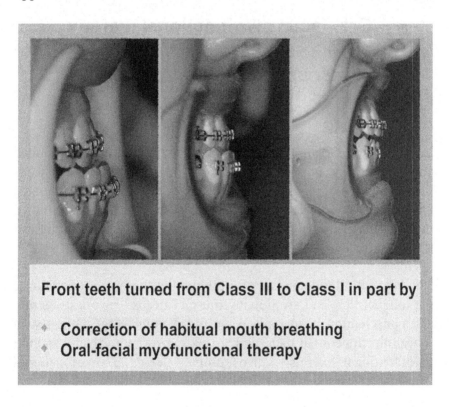

Front teeth turned from Class III to Class I in part by

- **Correction of habitual mouth breathing**
- **Oral-facial myofunctional therapy**

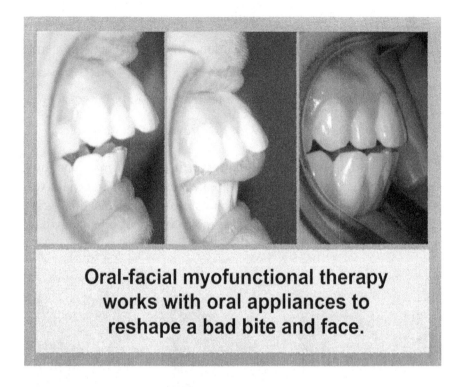

Oral-facial myofunctional therapy works with oral appliances to reshape a bad bite and face.

In short, orofacial myofunctional therapy trains the tongue and swallowing muscles to complement oral appliances' work on redeveloping the maxilla, the mandible, and the associated hard tissues. When tongue-tie is properly diagnosed, orofacial myofunctional therapy as a part of Holistic Mouth Solutions can keep your face looking younger despite gravity and time.

The key with the diagnosis of a tongue-tie: the owner-operator of the tongue, lips, and swallowing muscles needs to work diligently and conscientiously to replace the old dysfunctional pattern with a healthier functional pattern. This takes a lot more than watching myofunctional exercise videos online. Seeing a myofunctional therapist can be most helpful.

Holistic Mouth Bites

- The tongue is a major architect of your face and smile, but conditions such as tongue-tie and habitual mouth breathing can ruin their naturally beautiful design and initiate Impaired Mouth Syndrome.

- Laser release of tongue-tie followed by oral-facial myofunctional therapy has been shown to improve a long list of health problems and dental complications.

- Soft tissues shape the bones. If genes are not fully expressed, jaw structures do not reach their full potential, triggering a cascade of health problems.

- Orofacial myofunctional therapy is invaluable for correcting orofacial habits caused by tongue-tie—a condition with serious long-term consequences if left untreated.

Chapter Fourteen

Tongue-Tie's Treachery on Immune Health: Case Study

Oral diseases and conditions are related to other health problems.

– Oral Health in America:
A Report of the Surgeon General[1]

Tongue molding happens when a normal tongue is free to reach the roof of the mouth to serve as a natural palatal expander. This tongue molding results in a wider U-shaped palate. When I see a narrower V-shaped maxilla, I suspect tongue-tie, habitual mouth breathing, or both.

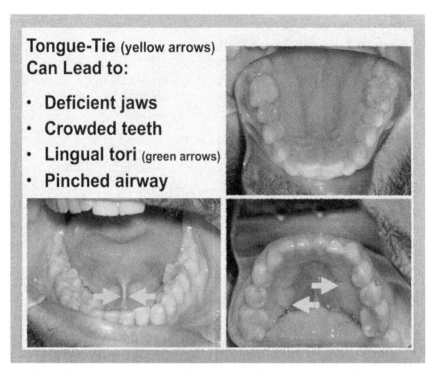

Tongue-Tie (yellow arrows)
Can Lead to:

- **Deficient jaws**
- **Crowded teeth**
- **Lingual tori** (green arrows)
- **Pinched airway**

C.K.'s tongue-tie (lower left), deficient maxilla (upper right), and lingual tori (green arrows) indicating chronic jaw clenching and teeth grinding.

While serious cases like Lucy's are starting to get the deserved attention early, milder cases of tongue-tie often go undetected, which can start a domino of medical-dental problems.

C.K. was born with a tongue-tie but did not find that out until he was forty-three and recovering from cancer. This is not to say that tongue-tie caused his cancer. There is no evidence for that yet. However, there is plenty of evidence linking airway obstruction to America's leading causes of death, including cancer.

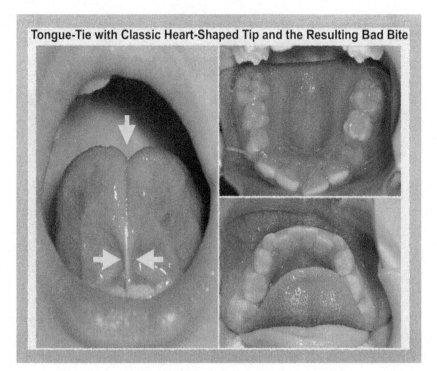

*Tongue-tie in a 9 year-old leads to narrow palate
and crowded lower front teeth.*

"About 28 million Americans have some form of sleep apnea," reported *The New York Times* in 2012, "though many cases go undiagnosed…. In one of the new studies, researchers in Spain followed thousands of patients at sleep clinics and found that those with the most severe forms of sleep apnea had a 65 percent greater risk of developing cancer of any kind."[2]

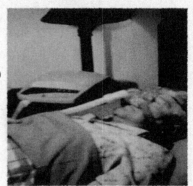

"Sleep-disordered breathing is associated with increased cancer mortality."
F. Javier Nieto and others, *American Journal of Respiratory and Critical Care Medicine* 186, no. 2 (2012): 190–194.

Adjusted Relative Hazard Ratio:

◆ 1.1 if Mild SDB   (AHI 5-14)

◆ 2.0 if Moderate SDB   (AHI 15-30)

◆ 4.8 = Severe SDB   (AHI > 30)

Mouth doctors are in a position to see oral-facial signs of airway obstruction early on.

Moderate OSA patients (AHI 15 to 30) had twice the risk of dying (mortality) compared to those with the same cancer but without OSA, while severe OSA patients (AHI above 30) had 4.8 times the risk, reported a twenty-two-year follow-up to the Wisconsin Sleep Cohort Study: "Baseline SDB [sleep-disordered breathing] is associated with increased cancer mortality in a community-based sample."[3]

Left unrecognized, tongue-tie is an oral condition that casts a very long shadow on health and life quality.

Tongue-Tie's Domino Effects: The Case of C.K.

C.K. had just finished chemotherapy for testicular cancer when he first came to see me. "My doctor-wife says she can't fix me by herself and that I need to see you."

"Your doctor-wife is a real integrative doctor. So tell me, if Fairy Godmother could wave away your top three symptoms you're living with now, which ones would you ask of her?"

"First, get rid of my cancer, of course," he said. "Then tiredness on waking up, sleepiness during the day, major brain fog, feeling winded, and leg edema and neuropathy."

"That helps me understand you better. Some of these are chemo-related, of course, but not all. When was the last time you had a good week's sleep?"

"About four years ago—before our daughter was born."

"That's understandable. Let's take a look at your mouth."

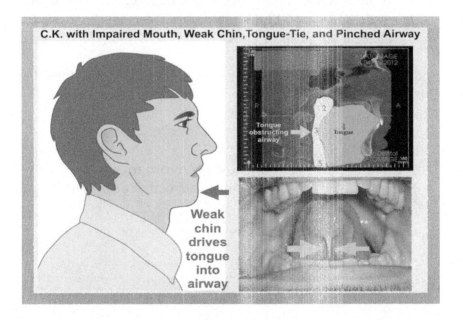

C.K. with Impaired Mouth, Weak Chin, Tongue-Tie, and Pinched Airway

Weak chin drives tongue into airway

Holistic Mouth checkup revealed:

- C.K.'s oral airway's narrowest diameter was only 30 percent of low normal.

- His nasal passage was mostly blocked. ("Yes, I have constant stuffy nose," he said.)

- He had crowded teeth with matching wear facets indicative of teeth grinding.

- His lower jaw had bony outgrowths on the tongue side called lingual tori, which are suggestive of jaw clenching and teeth grinding.

- He had tongue-tie.

- He had clicking jaw joints and jaw deviations on opening and closing his mouth (TMJD).

- His Epworth sleepiness score was 14 out of a possible 24, well above the low-risk range of 3 to 8.

- A sleep test confirmed teeth grinding, leg movement, and restless sleep of 17.8 sleep arousals per hour, but not the medical diagnosis of OSA.

Shortage of oxygen is a condition for cancer, according to Nobel Prize winner Otto Warburg, even if C.K.'s sleep test did not rule in OSA.

Bruxism and Leg Movements: C.K.'s Medical Diagnosis from Sleep Test

minutes. The total sleep time was 331.0 minutes. The patient spent 1.7% of total sleep tim N2, 20.2% in Stages N3 and N, and 32.0% in REM. Sleep latency was 24.4 minutes. RE Sleep Efficiency was 76.3%. Sleep Maintenance Efficiency was 80.9%. Total wake time wake percentage of 19.2%. 17 80.9

RESPIRATORY EVENTS: The polysomnogram revealed a presence of 0 obstructive, 3 resulting in an Apnea index of 0.5 events per hour. There were 4 hypopneas resulting events per hour. There were 29 RERAs rendering a RERA index of 5.3 per hour. The (Respiratory Disturbance) index was 1.3 events per hour.

Baseline oxygen saturation was 96.1%. The lowest oxygen saturation was 91.6%.

LIMB ACTIVITY: There were 40 limb movements recorded. Of this total, 14 were classi were associated with arousals. The Limb Movement index was 7.3 per hour while the PL

CARDIAC SUMMARY: The average pulse rate was 59.3 bpm. The minimum pulse maximum pulse rate was 100.0 bpm.

IMPRESSION: bruxism and leg movements' present, minimal respiratory disturbances

DIAGNOSIS: bruxism and leg movements

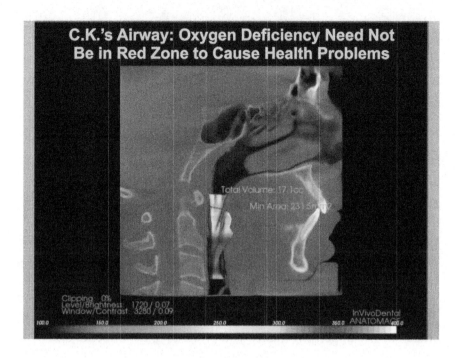

A "Lemon" Mouth's Systemic Effects

"Mr. K, if I may use a car analogy, you have a 'lemon' for a mouth. Were you breast-fed?"

"My mom tried, but she said I could not latch on."

"That's a red flag in my book. You have a pretty severe case of tongue-tie. Did you have lots of antibiotics in your early childhood?"

"Yes, I had lots of ear and sinus infections growing up. How can you tell?"

"I've seen this pattern many times: tongue-tie understandably leads to bottle-feeding, which in turn creates malocclusion—bad bite with crowded and crooked teeth from narrow and misaligned jaws."

"Oh? How?"

"Bottle-feeding and tongue-tie combine to create an abnormal swallowing pattern—picture a kid's mouth as they suck up a milkshake through a straw—which can lead to narrow jaws, crowded teeth, long faces, and very frequently a weak chin and clicking jaw joints."

"That's me alright. I also have frequent ear and sinus infections. Can they be connected to my mouth?"

Impaired Mouth's Role in Gut Inflammation and Allergies

"This is a common pattern I see, starting when an exhausted mom resorts to bottle-feeding to soothe the miserable baby with tongue-tie. This blocks full development, resulting in an impaired mouth, which is the structural start of snoring, sleep apnea, and teeth grinding later. Retruded jaws block the airway and disrupt sleep, and a narrow upper jaw makes you prone to sinus infections."

"That's why I had a lot of antibiotics and ear tubes as a kid and all my problems as a grownup?" C.K. asked.

"Yes. Now we know antibiotics can also kill good bacteria in the gut and create dysbiosis, in which bad bacteria dominate. German doctors know that life or death lies in the intestines. Improper weaning and premature introduction of adult foods then result in baby's gut inflammation." I continued, "This inflammatory bowel syndrome (often called 'leaky gut') can lead to food sensitivities, earaches, sinus infections, swollen tonsils, and a runny-stuffy nose that results in habitual mouth breathing, which then leads to oxygen deficiency, which leads to yet another way that an impaired mouth perpetuates gut problems."

"What's that?"

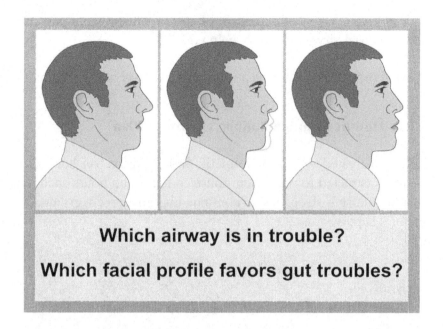

Which airway is in trouble?

Which facial profile favors gut troubles?

"Oxygen deficiency from an impaired mouth can aggravate dysbiosis, allergies, and fatigue in our adult years, all as a result of airway obstruction by the tongue."

"Yup, I've got major fatigue and gluten sensitivity and was finally diagnosed with celiac disease two years ago. I'm sure exposure to lots of fumes, chemicals, and vaccines in my military career didn't help."

"Health is the sum of many factors. Your tongue-tie didn't cause your cancer, but your mouth did put your health behind the proverbial eight ball long before you joined the military. It's fair to say your mouth is a big cause in your health's downhill slide."

"So what's your solution to my problem, doc?"

"Do you want to treat the symptoms or the causes?"

"My doctor-wife has said my cancer is a symptom. I want to get to the root causes because I sure don't want it back."

"I don't treat cancer, of course, but I can say this: opening up your oral and nasal airway can only help you."

"Let's fix my mouth then because I have a four-year-old daughter."

C.K.'s Holistic Mouth Solutions Treatment Plan

C.K. was treated with a biomimetic oral appliance on both jaws. He was instructed to wear them fourteen to sixteen hours each day, including during sleep, and to continue his cancer recovery under a doctor's supervision.

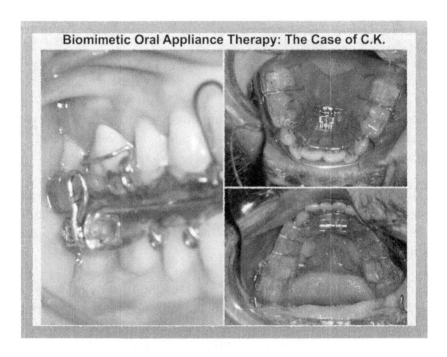

Biomimetic Oral Appliance Therapy: The Case of C.K.

C.K.'s Progress Report

After three months of wearing oral appliances to sleep and taking supplements from his doctor-wife, he reported being able to sleep through the night and having more energy during the day. "My attention and focus are getting better," he added.

C.K. is alive and well 5 years later, when I saw him at his doctor-wife's office party. While we don't know the conclusion to C.K.'s story, I believe his case does highlight two important points:

A. Tongue-tie can contribute to an impaired mouth, pinched airway, and eventually sleep apnea.

B. Tongue-tie is worthy of attention—and the earlier, the better.

Holistic Mouth Bites

- Tongue-tie can contribute to an impaired mouth, pinched airway, interrupted sleep, and a host of related health troubles. Research has shown that apnea and other sleep-disordered breathing appear to raise cancer risk.

- Breast-feeding is a crucial part of healthy orofacial development, letting the tongue do its work as a natural palatal expander.

- Unrecognized tongue-tie is all too often the first step in health's downward spiral. Releasing tongue-tie early is good proactive care.

Chapter Fifteen

Enjoying Freedom from CPAP: Case Study

Oftentimes, I recommend a referral to a dentist to treat obstructive sleep apnea. Most patients will ask me, "How is a dentist going to help me?" My answer is that since obstructive sleep apnea is mainly a problem from small jaws and crooked teeth, they have a variety of different ways of helping you to breathe better and sleep better.

– Steven Y. Park, MD,
Author of *Sleep Interrupted*[1]

"I can't get comfortable sleeping with a CPAP mask," said Robert, a fifty-eight-year-old gentleman at his first visit, "yet I know the importance of the airway and oxygen. Can I try an oral appliance instead?" He had been on a CPAP device for two years after a sleep test had diagnosed OSA.

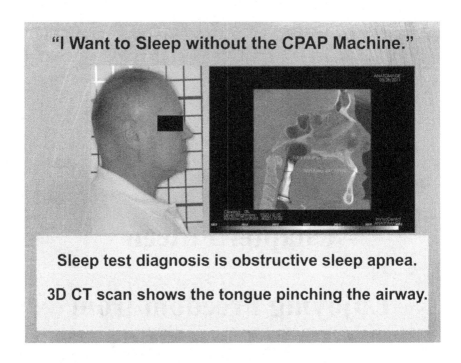

"I Want to Sleep without the CPAP Machine."

Sleep test diagnosis is obstructive sleep apnea.

3D CT scan shows the tongue pinching the airway.

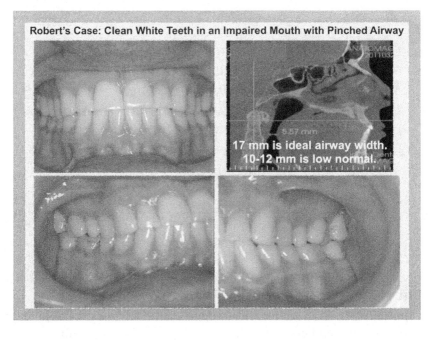

Robert's Case: Clean White Teeth in an Impaired Mouth with Pinched Airway

17 mm is ideal airway width.
10-12 mm is low normal.

At our initial consultation, Robert said his issues were daytime fatigue, needing a nap every day, annoying low back pain, and high blood pressure (140/90 where normal is less than 120/80). His Holistic Mouth checkup revealed good dental health with no cavities, nor gum disease, and:

- Medically diagnosed OSA with an AHI of 9.9 during REM sleep

- Low sleep efficiency at 79 percent, meaning he was not asleep 21 percent of the time he was in bed; his REM sleep was half of healthy normal at 16 percent.

- Mild forward head posture and posterior head rotation suggestive of airway deficiency

- Signs of teeth grinding, including generalized abfractions, gingival recession, and matching wear facets

- Mild to moderate crowding of his lower front teeth, suggesting a deficient maxilla

- A grade 4 Friedman tongue position (uvula not visible) suggests a high risk for OSA[2]

- An airway width of 5.57 mm at its narrowest on his 3D-CT scan, or less than half of low normal; his oral airway volume was 15.5 cc, about 40 percent less than comfortable.

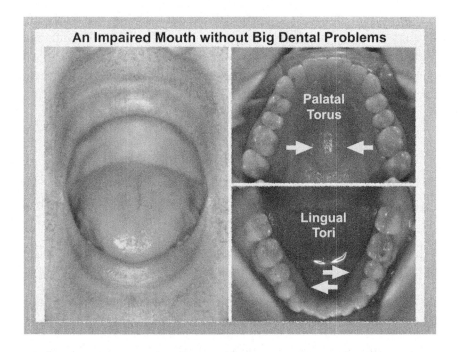

An Impaired Mouth without Big Dental Problems

Palatal Torus

Lingual Tori

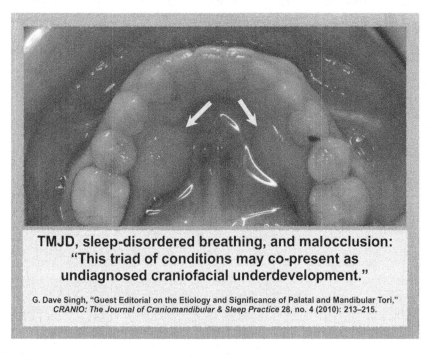

TMJD, sleep-disordered breathing, and malocclusion: "This triad of conditions may co-present as undiagnosed craniofacial underdevelopment."

G. Dave Singh, "Guest Editorial on the Etiology and Significance of Palatal and Mandibular Tori," *CRANIO: The Journal of Craniomandibular & Sleep Practice* 28, no. 4 (2010): 213–215.

I find this a very useful clinical pearl: "In adults, it is likely that palatal and mandibular tori are manifestations of undiagnosed sleep-disordered breathing, and may represent a valuable diagnostic sign in the triad of TMD, sleep-disordered breathing, and malocclusions."[3]

Cephalometrics showed a low ceiling for his "three-foot cage" and a Class III skeletal malocclusion—Robert's maxilla was retruded by 13 mm. The net effect was cramped quarters, forcing his tongue into his throat. This is how a retruded maxilla contributes to sleep apnea.

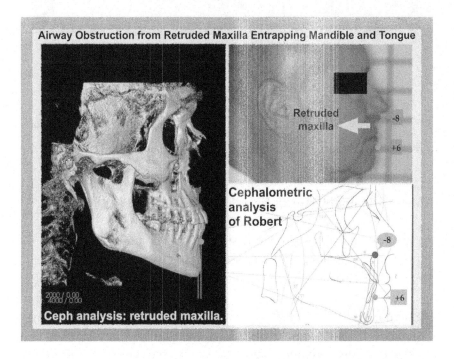

Ceph analysis: retruded maxilla.

Narrow Maxilla and OSA

If your paycheck is cut by 7 percent, do you feel it? The jaw width of OSA patients in Malaysia was found to be 7 to 11 percent narrower near the front of the upper dental arch, and 10-11 percent narrower in the molars region than non-OSA patients. "Supporting their role as etiological factors, size and shape differences in dental arch morphology are found in patients with OSA."[4]

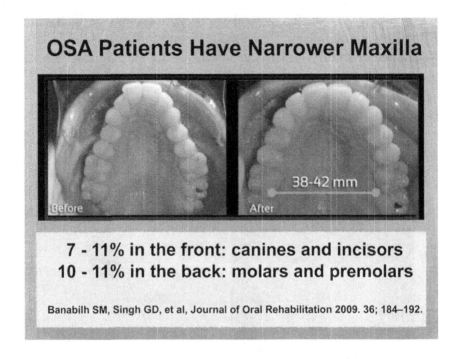

OSA Patients Have Narrower Maxilla

38-42 mm

Before After

7 - 11% in the front: canines and incisors
10 - 11% in the back: molars and premolars

Banabilh SM, Singh GD, et al, Journal of Oral Rehabilitation 2009. 36; 184–192.

Robert's Holistic Mouth Solutions Treatment Plan

At Robert's request to "keep it simple," we tried a mandibular oral appliance (OAm) first, but it failed to help his symptoms because his airway issue was rooted in his retruded maxilla.

He then opted for biomimetic (OAb) oral appliances. I used a type called an mRNA appliance, which combines maxilla treatment with mandibular advancement. We would redevelop his airway by epigenetically regrowing his maxilla in width, length, and height.

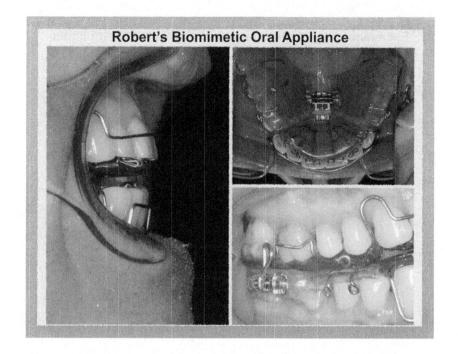

Robert's Biomimetic Oral Appliance

Robert was instructed to wear the appliance fourteen to sixteen hours a day, including during sleep, and turn the expander screw once a week. He was to see his own doctor and chiropractor as needed. I also provided sleep hygiene instructions: eat a small dinner at least four hours before bedtime; use blackout blinds in the bedroom; have no TV, cell phone, tablet, or computer there; and be in bed by 10:30 p.m. and asleep by 11 pm.

He would return once a month so that I could monitor his progress and adjust his bite as needed.

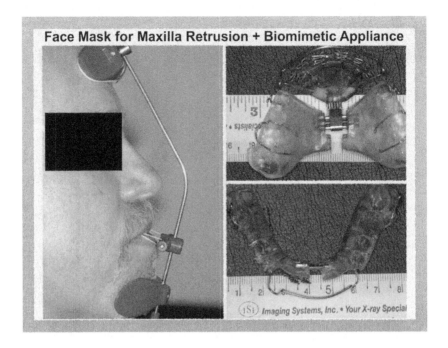

Face Mask for Maxilla Retrusion + Biomimetic Appliance

Results: CPAP Freedom

After a week of wearing the appliance, Robert said in a video for patients coming after him:

> *My name is Robert from Stafford, Virginia. I have had a week's time with the DNA appliance, both the upper and the lower. I had been using CPAP in the past and did not care for it at all. I did get some relief from my sleep apnea, but I do prefer the DNA device: less care with hoses and cleaning, and I am feeling quite refreshed. Don't need a nap in the afternoon like I did in the past. So if you are thinking of trying it, so far it's been a very positive experience for me.*

Over the course of two years, Robert made excellent progress. He gained 72 percent in his minimal airway width (9.56 vs. 5.57 mm) and 40 percent in airway volume (21.7 vs. 15.5 cc), and his jaw opening between the front teeth widened by 5 mm, indicating more relaxed jaw muscles. His Epworth sleepiness scale score dropped 47 percent, from 15 to 8, compared with the range of 0-10 in adults without a chronic sleep disorder.[5]

Robert then took a break from therapy for one year before resuming oral-appliance therapy. He made a second video two years from the start:

> *I continue to be very pleased with the decision. My energy level is much improved—no need for a nap in the afternoon, and no tossing around all night with that CPAP machine on. I would never go back to CPAP. Still using the appliance at night just to keep everything in place. If you are considering it, I would suggest looking at it as well.*

Robert understands sleep tests are needed down the road to monitor his OSA after oral appliance therapy is over.

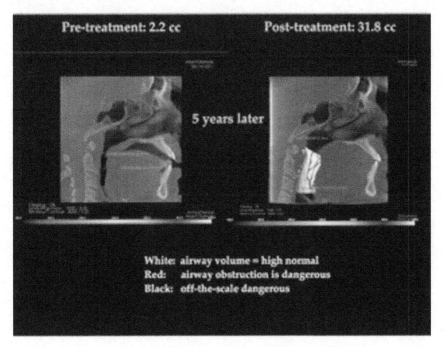

Both before and after images were taken without oral appliances in the mouth.

Biomimetic Oral Appliances: Airway Development without Surgery

The whole upper airway benefits from stem-cell activation by using a biomimetic appliance on the maxilla. A 2011 case report in *Dentistry Today* concluded, "Genetically encoded developmental mechanisms can be modulated by maxillary appliances to enhance the upper airway in adults."[6]

In my experience, biomimetic oral appliances are an effective solution to open up the airway while correcting the structural causes of crowded teeth, jaw-joint dysfunction (TMD), persistent pain, and chronic fatigue during sleep—provided that the patient actively changes their old habits and unhealthy lifestyle patterns. Robert certainly did.

Holistic Mouth Bites

- Biomimetic oral-appliance therapy can provide quick relief from sleep apnea in the short term while remodeling the airway over the long term in mild-moderate OSA cases.

- Robert's case illustrates how a pinched airway can be redeveloped in patients nearing 60 years of age as long as there are sound teeth and healthy gums.

- Fuller genetic expression can be achieved in the jaws and face using biomimetic appliances to redevelop both the maxilla and the mandible, as well as the airway.

Chapter Sixteen

Stem Cell Activation: The Natural Way to Airway Upgrades

The mouth reflects general health and well-being.

– Oral Health in America 2000:
A Report of the U.S. Surgeon General[1]

How does a biomimetic oral appliance upgrade an adult's airway? The short answer is stem cell activation. Here's a brief look into the science behind craniofacial redevelopment for adults.

Stem cells represent the latent ability to grow, adapt, repair, and regenerate. A baby grows from stem cells; so can underdeveloped jaws and a narrow airway, provided enough stem cells are available.

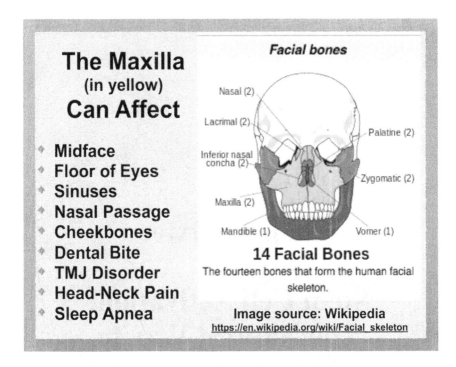

The Maxilla
(in yellow)
Can Affect

* Midface
* Floor of Eyes
* Sinuses
* Nasal Passage
* Cheekbones
* Dental Bite
* TMJ Disorder
* Head-Neck Pain
* Sleep Apnea

Facial bones

Nasal (2)
Lacrimal (2)
Inferior nasal concha (2)
Maxilla (2)
Mandible (1)
Palatine (2)
Zygomatic (2)
Vomer (1)

14 Facial Bones
The fourteen bones that form the human facial skeleton.

Image source: Wikipedia
https://en.wikipedia.org/wiki/Facial_skeleton

Sources of stem cells for craniofacial redevelopment include the tooth sockets in both jaws and jaw joints, and in cranial sutures, specialized joints by which the maxilla is connected to the face and head. Age is not a limiting factor, but the number of healthy teeth is.

Stem-cell technology means affected adults are no longer stuck with an impaired mouth structure and a pinched airway. As the maxilla redevelops in size, shape, volume, and position, the mandible is freed from its entrapment. As the three-foot cage between the jaws enlarges in volume, the pinched airway behind them also widens.

All this takes place without pain, simply by wearing a biomimetic oral appliance, and possibly an oral face mask, while you sleep. What a nice treatment!

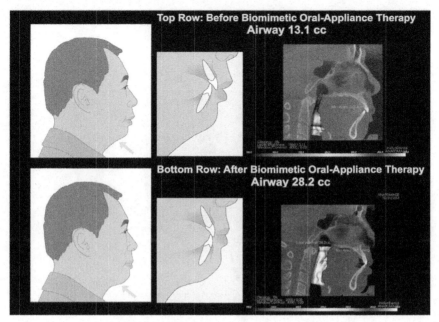

Craniofacial redevelopment using biomimetic oral appliance
more than doubles the airway in a man in his sixties.

Let's look deeper into the science behind biomimetic oral appliances.

Cranial Sutures: A Resource for Remarkable Results

Cranial sutures are specialized joints in the craniofacial skeleton that allow for the skull's slight movement which is essential for brain health. Sutures are important during growth and development and in allowing the skull bones to "breathe" in adults. This is called "cranial respiration" in the osteopathic field or "craniosacral rhythm" in the lay press.

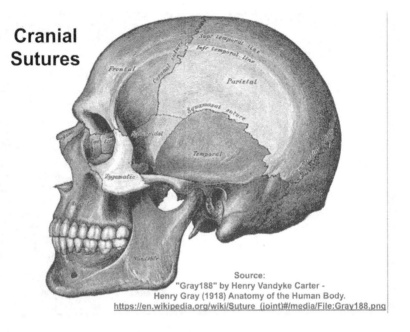

Cranial Sutures

Source:
"Gray188" by Henry Vandyke Carter -
Henry Gray (1918) Anatomy of the Human Body.
https://en.wikipedia.org/wiki/Suture_(joint)#/media/File:Gray188.png

The maxilla is connect to the cranium and face by seven sutures, which may not begin to fuse until 68-72 years of age, according to orthodontist Dr. Vincent G. Kokich in 1986, who postulated that adults "retain the capacity to regenerate and remodel bone at the craniofacial sutures."[2]

This means that the potential for maxilla-facial redevelopment is alive even late in adult life. My patients' experience agrees: age is not a limiting factor provided that there are enough healthy teeth.

Sutures have the potential to make bone: "Sutures are formed during embryonic development at the sites of approximation of the membranous bones of the craniofacial skeleton," reports a 2000 study in *Developmental Dynamics*."They serve as the major sites of bone expansion during postnatal craniofacial growth."[3]

In adults, this potential to make bone in the sutures surrounding the maxilla persists, because sutures may not close even late in adult life.[4]

Another study noted that "cells derived from normal and fused sutures displayed characteristics of the osteoblast [bone-forming] phenotype in culture."[5]

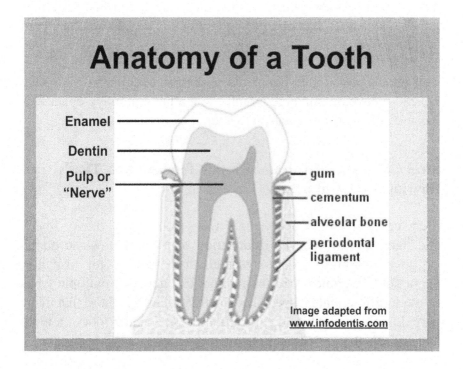

Anatomy of a Tooth

Enamel

Dentin

Pulp or "Nerve"

gum

cementum

alveolar bone

periodontal ligament

Image adapted from www.infodentis.com

The Surprising Common Feature of Periodontal Ligaments and Cranial Sutures

Periodontal ligaments anchor the teeth to the jaws. *Peri-* means around, and *-odontos* means teeth in Greek. Periodontal ligament exist in a 0.25 mm space that contains many interesting cells and sensors, including the ones that inform you of a bone chip in your burger, sand in your salad, or a shred of dental floss wedged between teeth.

Like cranial sutures, periodontal ligaments are both strong and elastic to absorb bite pressure. Dr. G. Dave Singh suggests that periodontal ligament spaces are actually a form of cranial sutures. "The periodontal ligament space is subject to sutural homeostasis, not unlike the sutures of the skull… Recent evidence suggests that this sutural width [of .025 mm] is tightly controlled at the genetic level."[6] "Most importantly," he adds, "it has been shown that the mammalian periodontium has a histologic structure that is akin to fetal tissues rather than mature adult tissues."[7] Fetal tissues are high in stem cells.

This means periodontal ligaments contain stem cells that can make bone to redevelop impaired mouth — another major eye-opener for me and one more great reason to keep up your dental health.

Stem Cells: The New Promise inside Tooth Sockets That's Blowing Away Old Beliefs

Stem cells in tooth sockets can make bone, gum tissue, fibers, and ligaments to keep the foundation of teeth (below the gums) in good working order. Research has shown, for instance, "periodontal ligament cell progenitors can generate multiple types of more differentiated, specialized cells", including those that make periodontal ligaments and cementum that covers the root of a tooth and embeds the periodontal ligaments.[8]

"Periodontal ligament fibroblasts after tooth extraction actively proliferate," notes another study. They "migrate into the coagulum, form dense connective tissue, and differentiate into osteoblasts which form new bone during socket healing."[9]

A 2004 NIH study similarly found that stem cells in the periodontal ligament expressed stem-cell markers. In other words, science has consistently shown the potential for stem cells in the periodontal ligament to create new bone and connective tissue.[10]

"Deep periodontal ligament cells retain the capability to differentiate into an osteoblast lineage [for making bone]." [11]. That means healthy teeth in sound jaw bone are needed for redevelopment.

Stem cells are only a promise. It takes a signal to flip on the switch and turn the promise into reality. The message is delivered in the form of a minimal stretch to the periodontal ligament that's felt as a a snugger fit of a special type of oral appliance. The message to the stem cells is: "Restart your bone-making assembly line that was once active during your teenage growth spurt that was mediated by your own genes."

When deficient jaws and a three-foot cage are redeveloped, the airway also widens, and sleep deepens. Growth hormones for repairing daily wear and tear are released only in deep sleep. This is a major outcome of Holistic Mouth Solutions.

From Promise to Reality: Biomimetic Oral Appliances

Biomimetic means to mimic natural biological processes of growth and repair. Biomimetics is a science that studies natural models and then uses these designs and processes to solve human problems, says Dr. G.D. Singh.

Biomimetic treatments are painless because they mimic (imitate) natural growth during teenage years. Biomimetic appliance is a new type of epigenetic oral appliance that can widen the airway and oral volume within the craniofacial skeleton to result in nonsurgical enhancement of the upper airway to relieve snoring and sleep apnea.

In theory, any maxillary appliance that can redevelop the deficient maxilla in adults and thereby free the mandible and tongue from entrapment has the potential to improve the upper airway. Available evidence shows that biomimetic appliances can remodel and widen an obstructed airway, so we will focus on them based on published evidence, while allowing that other types and approaches may also be effective.

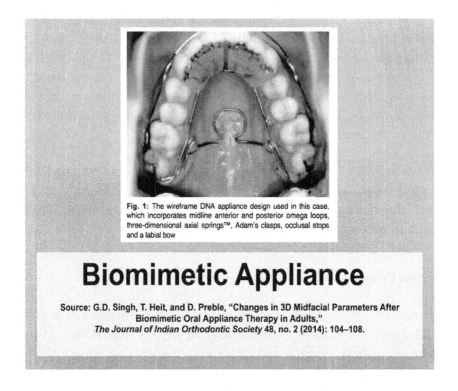

Fig. 1: The wireframe DNA appliance design used in this case, which incorporates midline anterior and posterior omega loops, three-dimensional axial springs™, Adam's clasps, occlusal stops and a labial bow

Biomimetic Appliance

Source: G.D. Singh, T. Heit, and D. Preble, "Changes in 3D Midfacial Parameters After Biomimetic Oral Appliance Therapy in Adults," *The Journal of Indian Orthodontic Society* 48, no. 2 (2014): 104–108.

Biomimetic Oral Appliance Therapy (BOAT): Evidence from Activating Stem Cells

Although epigenetic orthopedics is still in its infancy, evidence of biomimetic oral-appliance therapy's results is starting to come in. One study showed a 22 percent increase in the area behind the soft palate (the nasopharynx), a 16 percent increase in the area behind the tongue (the oropharynx). [12]

In a 2014 study, sleep test marker AHI dropped by 65.9 percent following biomimetic oral-appliance therapy (BOAT). "This preliminary study suggests that ... midfacial [maxillary] redevelopment may provide a potentially useful method of managing adults diagnosed with obstructive sleep apnea, using biomimetic oral appliances." [13]

A 2016 follow-up study showed a 64 percent drop in the AHI of severe OSA patients before and after BOAT. Conclusion: "BOAT may be a useful method of managing severe cases of OSA in adults, and represents an alternative to CPAP and MAD's [mandibular advancement devices]." [14] So BOAT has potential to treat severe OSA cases.

Epworth sleepiness scores decreased by 51.4 percent after BOAT, from an average of 8.2 ± 6 to 4.2 ± 3.6, in a 2016 *Journal of Dental Sleep Medicine* poster report I conducted with Dr. Singh. [15] Recall that the average Epworth sleepiness scale is 4.6 with a range of 0-10 in normal subjects. [16]

Taken all together, there is solid science behind Holistic Mouth Solutions using biomimetic oral-appliance therapy to redevelop the pinched airway inside underdeveloped jaws Now you can be free of that pinched airway and impaired mouth that have been bothering your sleep night after night and undermining your health year after year.

Holistic Mouth Bites

- Stem cells represent the latent ability to grow, adapt, repair, and regenerate. A baby grows from stem cells. Stem-cell technology means affected adults are no longer stuck with an impaired mouth structure and a pinched airway.

- Biomimetic oral appliances work by signaling and waking up stem cells in the tooth sockets, the sutures around the maxilla, and inside the jaw joints. This turns on the teenage growth spurt that was mediated by your own genes to grow bone in adults and transform an impaired mouth and pinched airway to a Holistic Mouth with a wider airway.

- A growing body of studies show that biomimetic oral appliances are effective for increasing oral airway width and volume, as well as alleviating OSA, making it a viable alternative to CPAP.

Chapter Seventeen

Promoting Children's Holistic Mouth Development and Full Genetic Expression

Pediatric obstructive sleep apnea in non-obese children is a disorder of oral-facial growth.

– Drs. Yu-Shu Huang and Christian Guilleminault[1]

Whole body health depends on a good night's sleep, which requires an unobstructed airway inside a fully developed face and jaws. A little oxygen deficit night after night adds up to a whole body bankruptcy decades later, as we have seen.

Lessons learned from treating adults with impaired mouths can be applied to keep children from suffering the same medical and dental troubles. This finding from pediatric sleep-apnea research indicates the importance of looking out for that six-foot tiger in a three-foot cage: "Persistent oral-facial problems were **always** identified as the prominent factor associated with failure to achieve a complete cure of OSA" [emphasis added].[2]

Prevention is in the dental profession's DNA. A Holistic Mouth checkup can screen for an impaired mouth and steer it in the right direction starting early in childhood.

Epigenetics: Environmental Factors Shaping the Jaws and Face

Two-thirds of the face is framed by the maxilla and the mandible, and the face you now have is the combination of your genes and epigenetics. (*Epi-* means "on top of".) "Epigenetics encompasses all processes that lead to heritable changes in gene expression without changes in the DNA sequence itself."[3]

My translation: epigenetics are non-gene factors that can influence developmental outcomes without changing the genes. Diet and exercise can change your health and body shape, but you'd have the same genes.

So what makes craniofacial development fall short in children to cause crowded teeth and "three-foot cage" in adults? Something else at work besides genes, and that's where epigenetic comes in.

In my experience, the top four most frequently overlooked epigenetic blockers to normal dental-facial development are tongue-tie, improper weaning, nasal congestion from environmental or dietary sources, and habitual mouth breathing. Others can include pacifiers, processed foods, antibiotics overuse, and "man-made sources like medicines or pesticides" according to the National Human Genome Research Institute.[4]

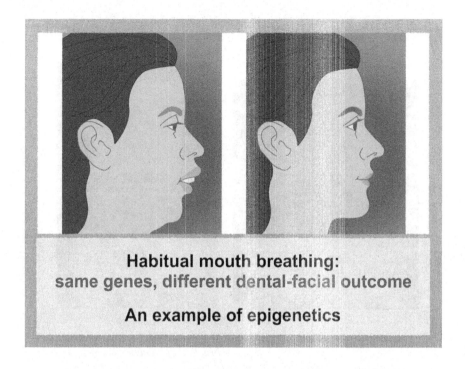

Habitual mouth breathing:
same genes, different dental-facial outcome

An example of epigenetics

Epigenetics can be applied just for a positive outcome as well, in my view. That's the aim of Holistic Mouth solutions. Early recognition and correction of tongue-tie and habitual mouth breathing are critical for Holistic Mouth development.

What Pediatric Sleep-Apnea Research Really Reveals

Pediatric OSA was first reported in 1976 by Dr. Christian Guilleminault, who noted that "subjects had narrowing behind the base of the tongue and oral-facial anatomical abnormalities."[5]

Historically, taking out enlarged tonsils and adenoids was the first treatment for pediatric OSA. Follow-up research showed that while surgery did improve sleep-test scores, only 27.2 percent had complete resolution of pediatric OSA.[6] In other words, for more than 70 percent of pediatric OSA cases, tonsils and adenoids surgery is not the final answer. So what is missing?

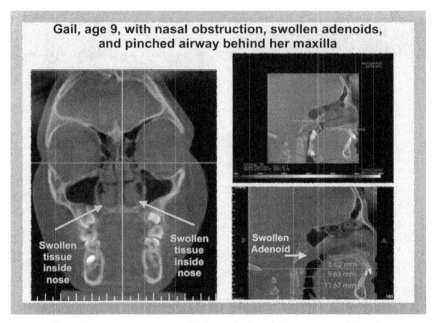

Gail, age 9, with nasal obstruction, swollen adenoids, and pinched airway behind her maxilla

Green arrows point to marked nasal obstruction as seen from the front. The gray is tissue while the black is air. The yellow arrow in the lower right image points to a swollen adenoid, which had closed down the nasopharyngeal airway by over 50 percent.

Fast-forward forty years, and we see that deficient jaw structure is the anatomical origin of OSA in newborns. According to Dr. Huang's 2015 study of 300 children in Taiwan, "Documentation of a high and narrow hard palate at birth predicts the presence of abnormal oral-facial features existing from birth in most cases [82 percent]." Further, "Only 9 percent of subjects … had a completely normal hard palate, normal breathing during sleep, and normal development."[7]

Dr. Huang's finding is strikingly similar to a 1955 osteopathic study by Dr. Viola Fryman who found 88 percent of participants had detectable cranial strains (twisted skull bones) at birth. Only 11.6 percent of newborns come through the birthing process with their soft skull bones holding alignment.[8]

"Considering knowledge accumulated since the 1970s on risk of abnormal maxilla and mandibular growth with abnormal breathing," concluded a 2013 study by Dr. Guilleminault, "regular follow-up of children with positive history of SDB should be performed particularly during oral–facial growth."[9]

In summary, deficient maxilla development and weak orofacial muscle tone lead initially to sleep apnea in children, and epigenetic airway redevelopment should pay attention to both hard and soft tissues.

An Ounce of Prevention: Holistic Mouth Checkup from Birth through Teens

A Holistic Mouth checkup starts with tongue-tie on the mouth floor and the airway in the nose and the back of the mouth. Seeing just the smile misses "the whole forest".

In my opinion, every newborn should be checked for tongue-tie, and a child should have a Holistic Mouth checkup as soon as they can cooperate with an evaluation, but no later than age eight. Left undetected, children with tongue-tie can grow into adults with problems stemming from "six-foot tiger inside a three-foot cage" problems.

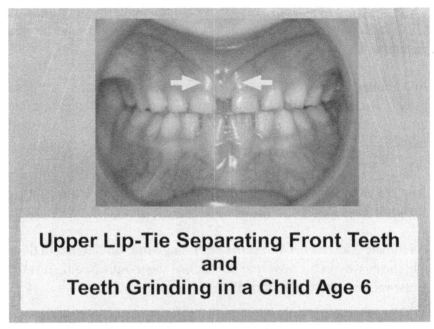

Upper Lip-Tie Separating Front Teeth
and
Teeth Grinding in a Child Age 6

Lip-tie will keep the front teeth separated, even after
braces, if left unrecognized and untreated.

Impaired Mouth Syndrome in children can include such signs and symptoms as habitual mouth breathing, stuffy/runny nose, hyperactivity, tiredness, grumpiness, teeth grinding, crowded teeth, bad bite (malocclusion), and more. Dr. Aelred Fonder found malocclusion to be a source of pains, more sinus infections, and underachievement in school. [10]

Bad Bite in High School Kids
Means More Pain + Infections

Source: Fonders AE, Dental Distress Syndrome Quantified, (1987) *Basal Facts*, 9(4), 141-167.

	Bad Bite	Normal Bite
⟡ Headaches	52%	22%
⟡ Facial Pain	84%	7%
⟡ Neck-Shoulder Pain	70%	48%
⟡ Backaches	65%	33%
⟡ Chronic Sinusitis	65%	30%
⟡ Acute Sinusitis	15%	0%

Less obvious tongue-ties that do not dramatically affect breast-feeding often lead to abnormal swallowing patterns, bad bite, and facial imbalance. In these borderline cases, a Holistic Mouth checkup can keep many subsequent medical, dental, and mood symptoms at bay.

The earlier the Holistic Mouth checkup, the better. "Every orthodontic case started after age 12 is a compromise," says Dr. Jay Gerber, longtime director of the Center for Orthodontic Studies. Dr. Gerber emphasized the pediatric airway as a maker of orthodontic success or relapse long before epigenetic studies emerged. My patients and I are beneficiaries of his teaching.

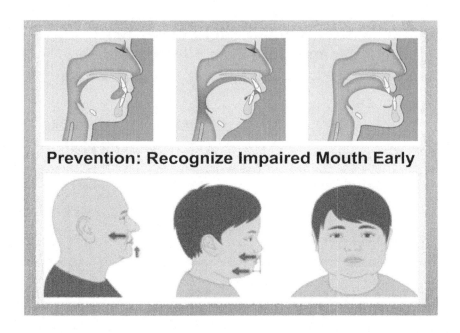

Human jaw and face development takes fourteen to eighteen years. By age twelve, the window of opportunity for fundamental correction is much smaller, especially if dental and facial development has resulted in a long face, a high and narrow palate, an excessive or weak chin, or a flat midface.

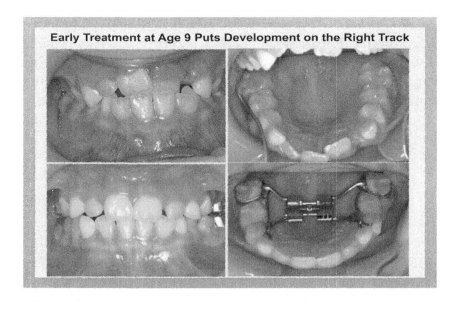

Freedom from the Perils of Habitual Mouth Breathing

In addition to tongue-tie, habitual mouth breathing is another serious epigenetic blocker of normal craniofacial-dental development.

"The airway functions, in a real sense, as a keystone for the face. The entire facial complex participates in the growth process. All parts and bony surfaces are involved. ... All are necessarily interrelated, and the developmental positioning, shaping, and sizing of any one part affect all others," notes Dr. Donald Enlow in *Handbook of Facial Development.* [11]

Failing to recognize habitual mouth breathing has serious developmental consequences. "All children who are habitual mouth-breathers will have a malocclusion," says Dr. John Flutter, a general dentist who practices orthodontics and orofacial orthopedics full-time in Brisbane, Australia. "Establishing nasal breathing in growing children must be a priority to prevent abnormal growth and development of the face and jaws. Establishing a lip seal in growing children must be the second priority." [12] I heartily agree.

There's plenty of evidence supporting this view, such as:

- A study published in *American Journal of Orthodontics* titled *Mouth Breathing in Allergic Children* reported: "mouth breathers' maxillas and mandibles were more retrognathic [retruded]. Palatal height was higher, overjet was greater in mouth breathers. Overall, mouth breathers had longer faces, with narrower maxillae and retrognathic jaws." [13]

- Earlier research in that same journal found that "all experimental animals [with artificially induced nasal obstruction or interference with lip seal] gradually acquired a facial appearance and dental occlusion different from those of the control animals." [14]

- A *CHEST Journal* study observed that "nasal congestion from any cause predisposes to sleep-disordered breathing." [15]

Optimal dental-facial form develops naturally through normal oral functions such as suckling, swallowing, chewing, and lip seal. As mentioned in chapter 13, "According to Moss, the form of the facial skeleton is largely secondary and adaptive to surrounding soft tissues and functional spaces." As the baby's brain grows, the cranial sutures respond to the subtle stretch by expanding the brain case.

Similarly, a perfectly suited functional space, for the tongue comes from normal soft-tissue actions of the tongue and the throat muscles on the inside, and lips and cheeks on the outside. This is how the genetic potential unfolds.

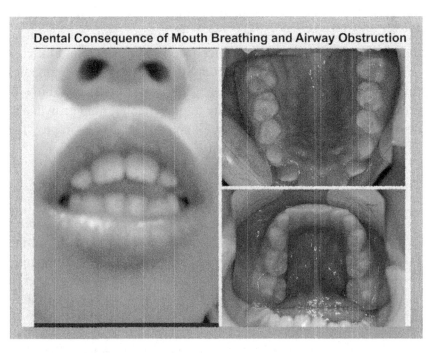

Would this child perform better at school from having a more open airway? Yes, I believe.

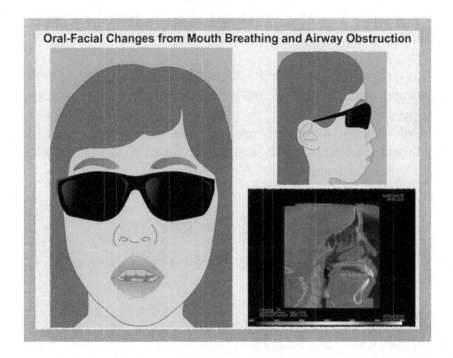

Oral-Facial Changes from Mouth Breathing and Airway Obstruction

Mouth breathing, like tongue-tie, interferes with the full expression of genetic potential. It can also lead to undesirable craniofacial changes. "The [breathing] impaired group demonstrate characteristic combinations of craniofacial deformities and malocclusions, with the younger individuals demonstrating a lesser expression of malocclusion progression and morphologic deformities," reports one 1988 study out of Case School of Dental Medicine. "This suggests that early recognition of such facial patterns may be utilized to identify those breathing compromised individuals who have a likely tendency to develop certain types of malocclusion." [16]

It's time to look beyond cavities and smiles in dental checkups. It's time for Holistic Mouth Checkups to uncover Impaired Mouth Syndrome early on to head off its devastating consequences later in life.

How Parents Can Monitor Their Children's Dental-Facial Development

Why do jaws become underdeveloped? Beyond tongue-tie, improper weaning, nasal congestion, and habitual mouth breathing, additional epigenetic factors can include prolonged bottle-feeding, pacifiers, thumb-sucking, a pro-inflammatory diet, exposure to industrial pollutants, maternal health and pelvic form, birth trauma to the skull, and accidental falls. [17, 18, 19, 20, 21, 22]

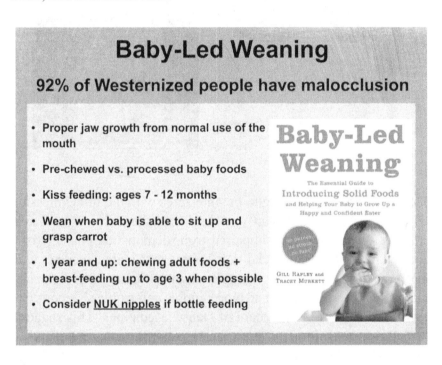

Why do teeth crowd up in children so frequently these days? It's not entirely the fault of the mom's or dad's genes. As Dr. Pottenger's famous studies of cats showed, a diet of processed foods can result in dental-skeletal malformation injuries that are passed down to offspring. "If proper nutrition and exercise are absent when facial structures are developing," he wrote, "dentition always suffers. The kitten kept on a deficient diet for 10 months has an inadequate jaw with crowded, irregular, and poorly aligned teeth." [23]

If nutritional injuries can lead to malocclusion and scoliosis, then can children with impaired mouth development be recipients of cumulative epigenetic patterns passed down from their family trees?

Ancestral diet has helped all ethnic groups survive to this day, but convenient food may be de-evolving the human dental-facial structures. This may explain the rise of malocclusion in children and the prevalence of sleep apnea and Alzheimer's disease in adults in Westernized countries. Much research is needed.

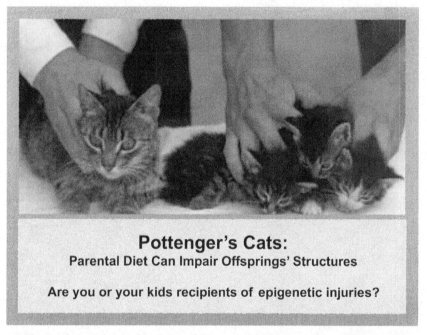

Pottenger's Cats:
Parental Diet Can Impair Offsprings' Structures

Are you or your kids recipients of epigenetic injuries?

The mother and grandmothers of these newborn kittens were fed a diet of cooked instead of raw meat; the kittens have dental-skeletal malformation.

Before all the studies are completed, there are constructive steps parents can take to guide their children's orofacial development onto the right track.

As always, parents should seek advice from their own doctors and dentists, as the information provided here does not constitute medical or dental advice.

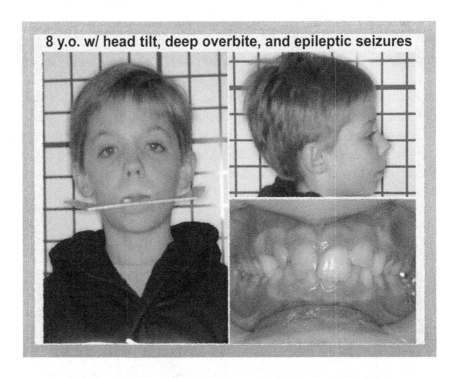

8 y.o. w/ head tilt, deep overbite, and epileptic seizures

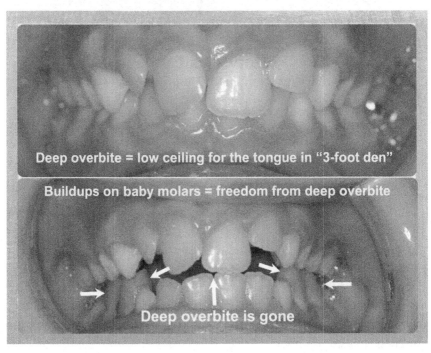

Deep overbite = low ceiling for the tongue in "3-foot den"

Buildups on baby molars = freedom from deep overbite

Deep overbite is gone

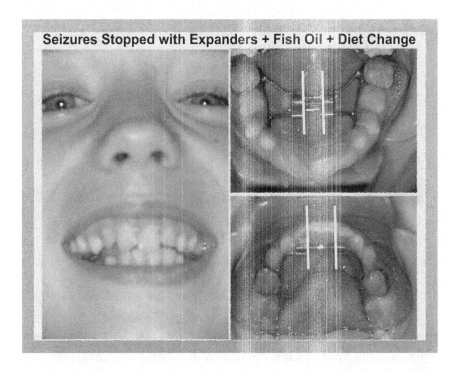

Seizures Stopped with Expanders + Fish Oil + Diet Change

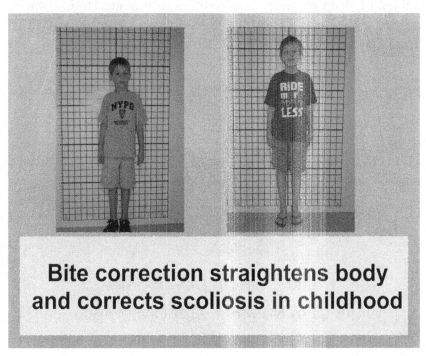

Bite correction straightens body and corrects scoliosis in childhood

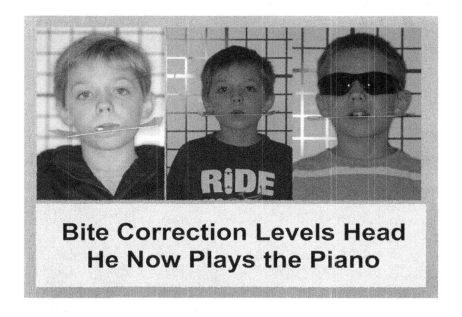

**Bite Correction Levels Head
He Now Plays the Piano**

Left undetected, impaired mouth development can lead to costly consequences later in adult life just on the dental side alone. Dentists trained in sleep medicine and certified to provide Holistic Mouth checkups can be a great asset to the cause of optimal orofacial development.

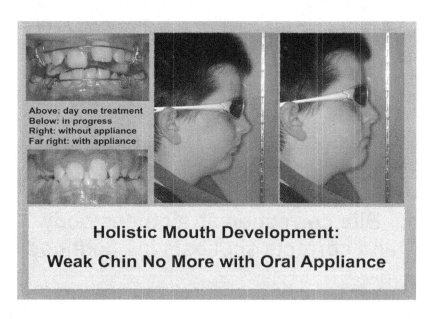

Above: day one treatment
Below: in progress
Right: without appliance
Far right: with appliance

**Holistic Mouth Development:

Weak Chin No More with Oral Appliance**

A Holistic Mouth checkup in early childhood is the best prevention of OSA and its complications. This requires integrative collaboration by all health professionals, parental awareness of Holistic Mouth connections, and additional training for interested dentists to see the whole mouth instead of just the teeth and gums.

A Parents'Guide to Holistic Mouth Development and other resources are available in the back of this book and at HolisticMouthSolutions. com.

Holistic Mouth Bites

- Tongue-tie, improper weaning, food sensitivities that can cause nasal congestion, and habitual mouth breathing are four commonly overlooked epigenetic blockers to normal dental-facial development, in my experience.

- The tongue inside the mouth, the nasal airway, and other soft tissues around the mouth shape the oral-facial structures. Poor soft-tissue function is the origin of impaired mouth development, airway obstruction and related consequences.

- Every newborn should be checked for tongue-tie, and a child should have a Holistic Mouth checkup as soon as they can cooperate with an evaluation, but no later than age eight.

- Crowded teeth, absence of lip seal, and habitual mouth breathing are signs of impaired mouth developing during childhood, and contributors to Impaired Mouth Syndrome in adult years.

Chapter Eighteen

The High Cost of Impaired Mouth: Two Cases and a Contrast

You see only what you know.

– Dr. Richard Beistle, DDS

One Dental Trouble After Another: The Case of Avis

"I have all conditions in that slide except high blood pressure," said 63-year old Avis, pointing at the image below. She had come in for an initial consultation regarding two other dental treatment plans totaling $29,000 and $19,000, respectively. Let's see if her dental troubles are connected to her medical symptoms through her impaired mouth.

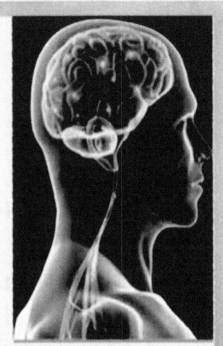

Impaired Mouth Often Comes With:

- Sensitive and high maintenance teeth
- Gum recessions
- Bladder urgency
- Morning headaches
- Daytime sleepiness
- Aches and pains, fatigue
- Pot belly, double chin
- Brain fog, poor memory
- Depression, anxiety
- Heart disease, high blood pressure

Holistic mouth doctors can evaluate and fix impaired mouth.

Avis kept her teeth and gums spotlessly clean. "But each time I go the dentist," she said, "there's something else wrong." Daily, she walked 5 to 7 miles for exercise, and she had lost weight since changing her diet. She had been doing her part, yet her teeth keeping having costly troubles. How could that be?

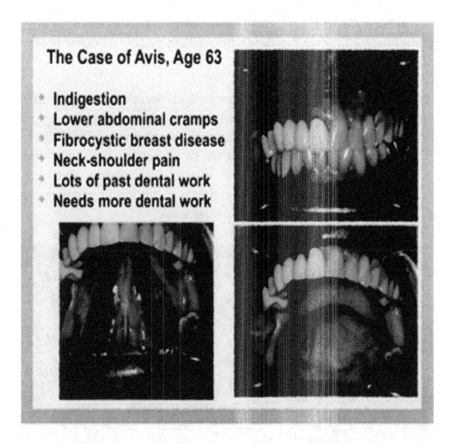

The Case of Avis, Age 63

* Indigestion
* Lower abdominal cramps
* Fibrocystic breast disease
* Neck-shoulder pain
* Lots of past dental work
* Needs more dental work

Our Chair Side Investigation revealed an important clue: Avis seldom woke up feeling refreshed – "less than twice a week since forever," she said. A 3D CT scan revealed an airway the width of angel hair (pasta). I gave her an overview of impaired mouth as a problem and Holistic Mouth as a solution. Then I asked her, "Would you mind telling me what you learned from coming to see me?"

"First, having a six-foot tiger in a three-foot den creates an airway issue. Secondly, airway comes before dental work."

"You've got it. Airway dictates, and the rest of the body adapts to a pinched airway by paying a price."

"I've been dealing with my teeth since my 20s. Even as they complimented me on my home care, I kept getting cavities, broken and root canal pain just the same."

"Poor dental hygiene is not your problem. Sleeping with a normal size tongue inside a half-sized mouth is. Each time you sleep, your body experiences an oxygen deficiency that threatens life. Oxygen deficiency results in higher acidity. To neutralize that acid, your body robs calcium from wherever it can, mainly bones and teeth. Another reaction to airway obstruction is teeth grinding, which can damage natural teeth and loosen dental work."

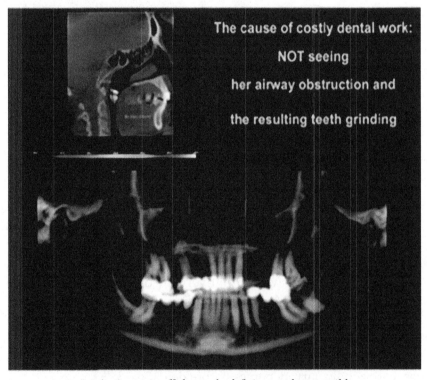

The cause of costly dental work:

NOT seeing

her airway obstruction and

the resulting teeth grinding

*Avis's airway is off-the-scale deficient and susceptible
to sleep apnea, thus hazardous to dental health.*

"Really?! That'd explain why I kept getting cavities over the past 30 years, even after I stopped all sweets. Apples and baked potatoes are the only treats I get. So where do I start?"

"You should still get your cavities treated to keep your teeth in good repair. But before your next dental reconstruction, let's fix your airway to avoid further damage from the same old pattern."

Avis frowned. "How come I never heard about Holistic Mouth before?"

"Dentists' eyes are trained to see teeth and gums. A mouth doctor looks at the airway, the neck, the jaw joints, the tongue space between the jaws. Airway blockage by the tongue starts as a mouth problem that creates teeth problems later. Here's the good new: you still have enough good teeth in the right places, and redeveloping your airway costs much less than a third of dental reconstruction."

"I can't wait to wake up feeling great for once in my life!"

The anatomical choke zones behind Avis' jaws is the source of her dental problem was also her medical problem, and Medicare's, and therefore all Americans'. What have her health insurance premiums and coverage gotten her? The patient has done her part, but has America's healthcare system?

The earlier the recognition and correction of impaired mouth, the lower the cost to individuals, employers, and Medicare.

The sensible sequence in building a house is to lay a foundation and frame the walls and floors before finishing the rooms and moving the furniture in. In the Old World mentality of dentists focusing on teeth, the furniture gets a makeover while the bad infrastructure is ignored and stays in trouble.

It is time to break out of the tunnel vision and see the airway as the starting point of dental care.

Having to Come Out of Retirement To Pay For Her Teeth: The Case of Marie

"The single greatest expense I have had for my health has been for my teeth." Marie was 62 one-retired but applying to go back to work when she came to see me. "I am here for a third opinion regarding my dental makeover. The price tags are $90,000 from one dentist, and $42,000 from another, and I cannot afford either."

Marie's presenting complaints included one dental problem after another since age 7, food sensitivity and gut inflammation, overweight, snoring, and her memory getting fuzzier. She had all the signs of an impaired mouth, including an extremely deep overbite, 10 crowns, 6 implants, and severe wear on her remaining teeth.

"I've been stationed all over the world, and I have seen at least 50 dentists in my life," Marie said. "None has ever told me why I grind my teeth or that my airway is a problem."

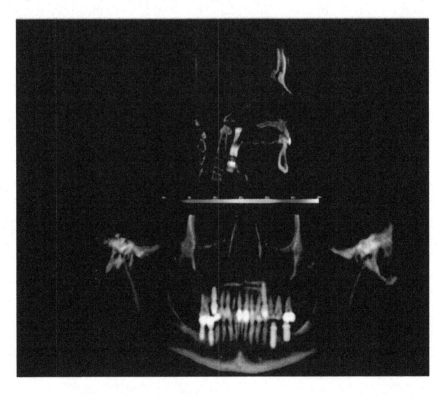

I referred Marie for a sleep test, and the medical diagnosis was moderate obstructive sleep apnea (AHI =18). Her lowest oxygen concentration dropped to 68%, whereas "healthy" is considered 95% or more. Left untreated, this has serious implications on brain function and memory.

"How's your adrenal function?" I asked.

"Oh, yes, my doctors are trying to fix that too."

"Sleeping with the tongue occupying your airway is like burning the candle from both ends. You're struggling to stay alive during sleep when you should be resting and renewing yourself."

"I can feel that first hand, but you're the first doctor who's ever said that to me."

"My work focuses on providing a more compatible space for your tongue so it's not forced into the throat. In building a house, the foundation and the framework should be in place before moving the furniture in, right?"

"Right. But all I'm getting so far is furniture replacement at an astronomical price, and it doesn't even address the root cause." Marie shook her head.

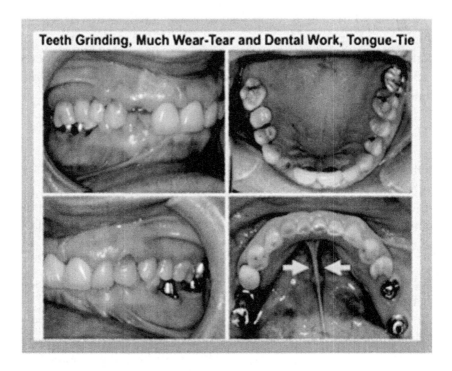

Teeth Grinding, Much Wear-Tear and Dental Work, Tongue-Tie

In my view, Marie's very deep overbite was a surface sign of her impaired mouth and pinched airway that was an anatomical source of nearly all her medical and dental troubles.

The dental diagnosis in Marie's case was Class I malocclusion with a strong deep bite tendency. But it said nothing about the cause and the logical treatment. So the dentists kept fixing the dental wear and tear, while her mouth had gone missing in her medical and dental care.

"You have a case of six-foot tiger inside a three-foot den with a very low ceiling and shallow depth front-to-back.," I explained to her, "The solution depends on your choice: Sleep with a CPAP machine or redevelop your jaws with oral appliances to free your lower jaw from its entrapment and liberate your tongue from the airway?"

"I don't want to sleep with forced air. I want to fix the cause," Marie said.

"In that case, airway comes before teeth. Before we can start, however, your case is complicated by pre-existing bridgework perpetuating your narrow airway."

"I see that now. So how do we start fixing my problems?"

"The size of your airway is determined by the combination of soft tissues excess (over-weight and nose-throat inflammation), and hard tissues (jaw size, position, and deep overbite). So the logical order for treating your case is to start with ensuring nasal breathing full-time and oral appliances to redevelop both jaws. You will still need to reconstruct your old bridgework, but only after your airway problem is solved."

"Now I definitely have to un-retire and go back to work!" she said with a smile.

Once patients know the cause of their troubles, most want to fix it. My heart goes out to Marie – and all patients who have had extensive dental work done while their OSA has gone undiagnosed. Until sleep and airway issues routinely turn up on a dentist's radar screen, healthcare costs will be high for patients stuck with undiagnosed impaired mouths, as well as their employers and our national treasury.

The Joys – and Cost Savings – of Childhood Holistic Mouth Development: The Case of S.B.

S.B. is the oldest of five children whose parents are members of the Weston A. Price Foundation and follow the Nourishing Traditions Diet. S.B. came in at age 11 with no cavities, strong teeth, and a good face. His mom was concerned with crowded teeth, cross bite in one tooth, and fang-like canines that did not fit into his upper arch.

A few months of oral appliance therapy amplified S.B.'s good genes and diet so that he did not need braces. His parents used the savings on oral appliance therapy for the younger siblings.

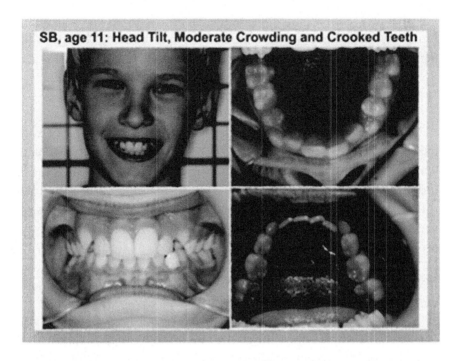

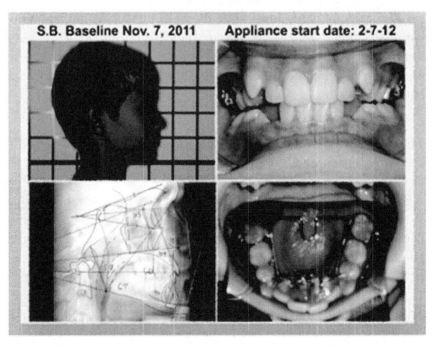

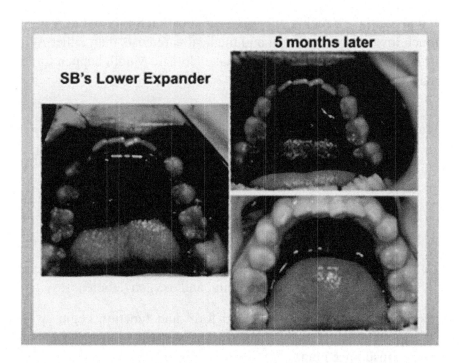

5 months later

SB's Lower Expander

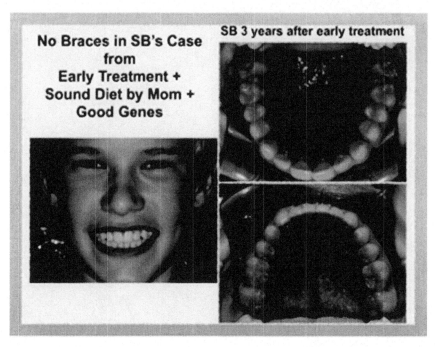

No Braces in SB's Case
from
Early Treatment +
Sound Diet by Mom +
Good Genes

SB 3 years after early treatment

It does not take a rocket scientist to predict that S.B. will likely have much lower lifetime dental and medical care costs than either Avis or Marie. Wouldn't it be nice to make Holistic Mouth happen for as many Americans as possible?

Holistic Mouth Bites

- The pattern of "one dental trouble after another" is a red flag for an impaired mouth. Very high dental and medical bills happen when the impaired mouth goes missing in medical care and the pinched airway goes missing in dental care.

- Airway before Teeth: redevelop impaired mouth as a root cause before spending lots of money rebuilding teeth damaged by acid reflux, teeth grinding, and oxygen deficiency.

- The U-turn back to sound form and function begins with a holistic mouth checkup and a more integrative health insurance plan.

Chapter Nineteen

The Holistic Mouth Checkup: Integrating Mind, Body, and Mouth

That it is important to correct perpetuating factors is illustrated by the apocryphal story of the man who stepped into a hole in the sidewalk and broke his leg. He was treated and the bones of his leg healed, but two months later he stepped in the same hole, and again broke the leg. **No one had patched the hole.**

– Myofascial Pain and Dysfunction: The Trigger Point Manual[1]

Impaired mouth is an unseen "hole in the sidewalk" in American health care today, and the vastly under-recognized Impaired Mouth Syndrome is costing every American medically, dental, and financially.

When all the research is done eventually, an impaired mouth is either an initiating or contributing factor in snoring, sleep apnea, nagging aches and pains, chronic fatigue, moodiness, lingering illness, and the puzzling and yet costly pattern of one dental problem after another. That's because the mouth belongs in the body's control tower, where it participates in essential functions such as breathing, sleep, energy, digestion, speech, socializing, relationship building, life quality, and longevity.

The whole body suffers when the mouth is structurally impaired, and so does the pocketbook. It's time to put Holistic Mouth Checkup to uncover Impaired Mouth as a handicap and reverse the Impaired Mouth domino with Holistic Mouth Solutions™.

Impaired Mouth: Hugely Expensive, Hugely Preventable

A Holistic Mouth Checkup has one purpose: to help you and your doctors determine if impaired mouth is a built-in stressor contributing to pain, fatigue, early degeneration, and to help parents prevent impaired mouth's systemic consequences for their children.

Todd, age 14, was referred by his mom's natural hormone doctor who suspected tongue-tie and its effects on airway and sleep. Mom's concerns included "slow to reach puberty, a lot of teeth grinding, and some ADHD. Otherwise he has been really healthy." Chair Side Investigation confirm the presence of tongue-tie, partial nasal obstruction, enlarged tonsils and adnoids, and a narrow airway in the red zone behind his palate.

Diagnosis: Impaired Mouth and pinched airway interfering with the start of puberty. His Holistic Mouth Solutions™ treatment included the following: diet change to ensure nasal breathing full-time, wear an upper oral appliance attached to a face mask to sleep for ten months, tongue-tie release, and oral-facial myofunctional therapy.

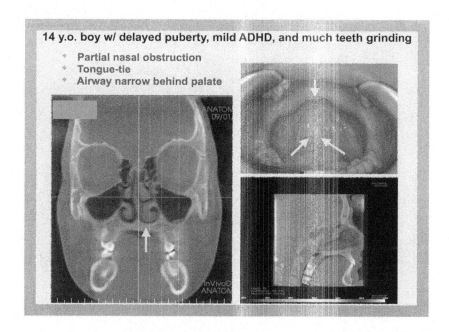

14 y.o. boy w/ delayed puberty, mild ADHD, and much teeth grinding
- Partial nasal obstruction
- Tongue-tie
- Airway narrow behind palate

"I wake up less tired, and I have more energy during the day compared to before starting oral appliance", says Todd 3 months later . (He goes to school many states away.) "I am proud of you for doing your part." I padded him on the shoulder, "But you can do more." Todd wore his oral appliance only during sleep, i.e. only half the recommended time, but it still worked. Todd agreed that he'd wear his appliance from after dinner to breakfast by signing his name on his chart.

Then I commented to Todd's mom, "His legs look longer to me." Yes, and Todd had just gotten bigger shoes and longer pants — evidence that growth spurt is kicking in. Coincidental? Maybe, maybe not. One thing is sure: growth hormones are released during deep sleep. Oral appliance therapy may jump-start delayed puberty through airway development and deeper sleep. A formal study is needed to confirm that opinion.

A positive domino effect starts Todd back on the right track with that referral by his mom's WholeHealth-oriented doctor. The resulting early intervention can save him many medical, dental, and other troubles throughout life, unlike the cases cited in the preceding chapters.

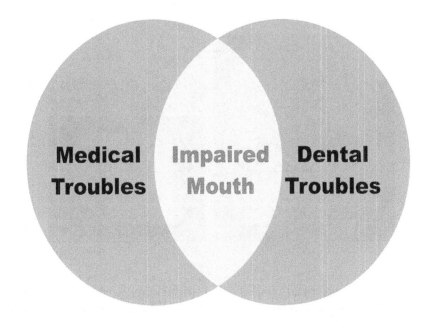

With training, all health professionals and even some patients can screen for an impaired mouth and recognized Impaired Mouth Syndrome. Dentists who are certified as Holistic Mouth doctors can confirm the presence of impaired mouth, screen for airway and sleep problems, refer for sleep test work with integrative health professionals as needed, and provide Holistic Mouth Solutions to help save teeth, hearts, money, and lives.

A patient's total health will upgrade itself naturally if a Holistic Mouth checkup is part of the medical and dental diagnostic process that results in treating the anatomical source of Impaired Mouth Syndrome.

A patient's total health can upgrade itself naturally only if sleep and airway is not blocked by an Impaired Mouth. Living and sleeping with an impaired mouth makes health a difficult and costly quest for patients, employers, insurance carriers, and the government. **Improving natural** health through sleep upgrade is an effective and sustainable way to reduce the cost of managing Impaired Mouth Syndrome.

More patients will be better served if more health professionals can:

1. Recognize the need for a Holistic Mouth checkup

2. Know how to screen for an impaired mouth

3. Have certified Holistic Mouth doctors to refer to for Holistic Mouth Solutions

4. Have the support of employers, insurance carriers, and government leaders in these endeavors as they do traditional dental checkups and cleanings

In this book, we have looked solely at the consequences of an impaired mouth on airway-related complications, which are already considerable. Medically, we've seen how impaired jaw development leads to obstructive sleep apnea (OSA), which is "a common but under-diagnosed disorder that is associated with excessive sleepiness, poor quality of life, neuro-cognitive deficits, metabolic dysfunction, cardiovascular disease, and early mortality," as one study in *JAMA* found.[2]

It is worth looking again at the leading problems stemming from OSA:

• Hypertension and heart failure

• High blood pressure, stroke, and heart attack

• Inflammation and oxidative stress

• Obesity-related ailments

• Alzheimer's disease

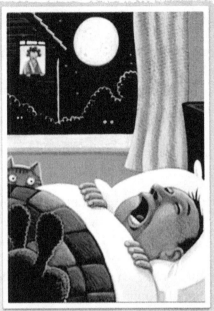

Obstructive Sleep Apnea (OSA) Symptoms:

- High blood pressure, stroke*
- Heart attack, sudden death*
- Diabetes, obesity*
- GERD: acid reflux*
- Lower immunity*
- Depression, anxiety*
- Brain fog, senile memory*
- Accelerated aging*
- Chronic pain*
- Daytime sleepiness, accidents*
- Sleep bruxing (Teeth grinding)

*William C. Dement and Merrill M. Mitler, *JAMA* 269, no. 12 (1993): 1548–1550.

Each of these conditions is expensive to live with—and to pay for. Unsurprisingly, the more severe the sleep apnea, the higher the medical cost.

Would the cost of disease management go down substantially if we treat impaired mouth as an anatomical root cause of poor sleep and oxygen deficiency? I believe the answer is definitely! Consider just Alzheimer's disease for a moment.

CDC research spells out just how big this problem is: "One in eight Americans aged 60 and over (12.7 %) say they have experienced worsening confusion or memory loss in the previous 12 months …. Of those experiencing worsening memory problems—known as 'cognitive decline'—over 80 percent have not talked to a health provider about it; and 1 in 3 says memory loss has interfered with household activities and/or work."[3]

Linda, age fifty-seven, recognizes her husband on some days, but not others. She had been the manager of a departmental store's cosmetic counters before she was diagnosed with Alzheimer's disease. Linda's first visit with me was a routine six-month cleaning, during which I found a mouthful of gum inflammation, which has been linked to Alzheimer's as well.[4] In addition, Linda had many fillings and crowns and a narrow V-shaped maxilla.

I sent her for a sleep test because she had never had one done. I told Linda's family that a 2009 preliminary study had shown that "sustained use of CPAP slows deterioration of cognition, sleep, and mood in Alzheimer's disease and obstructive sleep apnea."[5] As basic care, we are now waiting for Linda's son to arrange for help to supervise her home care to control her gum bleeding.[6]

With Baby Boomers now aging and retiring, says the Alzheimer's Association, "The rising costs of Alzheimer's disease are on a path that will cripple state budgets. A comprehensive strategy is needed."[7] We can no longer afford to ignore choked airways inside impaired mouths.

Supplying the brain with all the oxygen it needs, particularly during sleep, is a sensible start to reviving a brain undergoing cognitive and memory decline. Ruling out airway obstruction inside an impaired mouth is a logical, low-cost first step. "If only we could have had this cleaning with you ten years earlier," sighed Linda's husband.

Dentists Trained as Holistic Mouth Doctors Have a Strategic Position to Screen for OSA During Checkups

Given the primarily oral nature of OSA, dental visits make excellent opportunities for screening for OSA, fixing Impaired Mouth, and stopping the many costly related complications.

It's time to connect medical and dental symptoms with sleep and the airway and therefore impaired mouth structure. As mentioned in the Introduction, this holistic integration of mind-body-mouth is not part of health professionals' training. The earlier an impaired mouth is diagnosed, the lower the cost of managing obstructive sleep apnea and its related symptoms. Fatigue "since forever" is a recurring theme in my chair-side chats with new patients, as are aches and pains, snoring, and teeth grinding.

Total Health Benefits of a Holistic Mouth Checkup

The body's innate ability to heal and renew itself can be activated through deeper sleep by redeveloping an impaired mouth into a Holistic Mouth—one that is structurally fit to support total health. This requires a new breed of qualified mouth doctors who are trained on a postgraduate level.

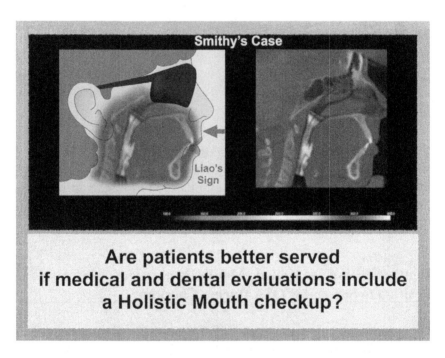

A dentist trained to provide a Holistic Mouth checkup can help patients and their doctors and all health professionals:

- Determine if the patient has an impaired mouth that results in a pinched airway

- Recognize the signs and symptoms of snoring, teeth grinding, and malocclusion

- Screen for sleep-apnea risk during regularly scheduled dental checkups to help reduce OSA-related co-morbidities in, around, and beyond the mouth

- Provide oral appliances and Holistic Mouth Solutions

- Collaborate with medical (and all health) professionals to treat patients who have mild to moderate OSA or who don't tolerate continuous positive airway pressure (CPAP) therapy

- Identify, mitigate, or resolve oral contributions to chronic pain and fatigue

- Educate patients on the need for lifestyle change, taste reform, and stress management

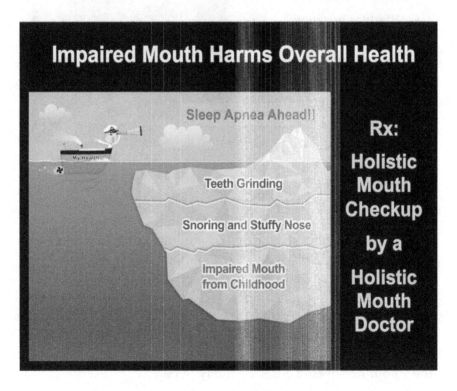

Reclaim Your Fully Potentiated Mouth and Health: Start by Having the Right Conversation with Your Health-Care Providers

If you have any of the signs and symptoms discussed in this book, I encourage you to start conversations with your medical, dental, and integrative health-care providers on how to avoid that "unpatched hole" that we have identified as an impaired mouth with a pinched airway.

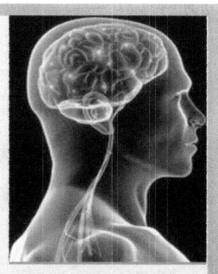

Impaired Mouth Often Comes with:

- Sensitive and high-maintenance teeth
- Gum recessions
- Bladder urgency
- Morning headaches
- Daytime sleepiness
- Aches and pains, fatigue
- Potbelly, double chin
- Brain fog, poor memory
- Depression, anxiety
- Heart disease, high blood pressure

Holistic mouth doctors can evaluate and fix impaired mouth.

Holistic Mouth checkups help ensure that you have the right infrastructure to supply oxygen without interruption to your heart, brain, and teeth that may already be starving for it.

The earlier your mouth impairments and airway obstructions are spotted and treated appropriately, the less frustrated you're likely to be with your health, the less pain you are likely to have, and the lower your health-care costs are likely to be.

The medical and dental worlds currently remain far too segregated for your whole-body health. As a patient, you can start the conversation about your sleep and airway with your doctors and dentists using this book, your Holistic Mouth score, and your Epworth sleepiness scale. I've included resources at the end of this book to support you in this endeavor, as well as a special section at HolisticMouthSolutions. com, giving you additional tools and support so that you can take charge of your health like never before.

Holistic Mouth Bites

- A Holistic Mouth checkup has one purpose: to help you and your doctors and health professionals determine if your mouth is a built-in stressor contributing to poor sleep, oxygen deficiency, and medical, dental, mental-emotional, and financial troubles.

- Dental visits are excellent opportunities to screen for an impaired mouth and OSA, as long as a trained Holistic Mouth Doctor is in.

- Natural health upgrade through better sleep and wider airway from Impaired Mouth recognition and Holistic mouth solutions can be an effective and sustainable way to reduce the cost of managing the "unmatched hole" of Impaired Mouth Syndrome.

- A Holistic Mouth checkup bridges the gap between the segregated medical and dental worlds. The earlier an impaired mouth and an obstructed airway are recognized and treated appropriately, the less pain the patient suffers and the lower the health-care cost.

Chapter Twenty

From Teeth to Mouth: Dentistry's Next Paradigm Shift

We are each other's harvest; we are each other's business; we are each other's magnitude and bond.

– Gwendolyn Brooks

At the end of each tooth, there is a whole person. I learned that in dental school.

At the end of each mouth, there is an airway that impacts medical, dental, and life quality, as well as out-of-pocket costs, insurance premiums, competitive edge, and taxes. I learned that from seeing patients as a mouth doctor.

Through these pages, we have seen the whole-body fallouts of an impaired mouth too small for the tongue—a six-foot tiger in a three-foot cage. This diagnosis also suggests its own solution: enlarge the tongue's habitat, and good sleep and energy will naturally follow.

Now let's turn to the next challenge: The mouth is still largely missing in American health care today. The waiting rooms of emergency rooms, hospitals, and doctors' offices are filled with patients suffering from symptoms of impaired mouths yet to be diagnosed. What will it take to turn this awareness into action?

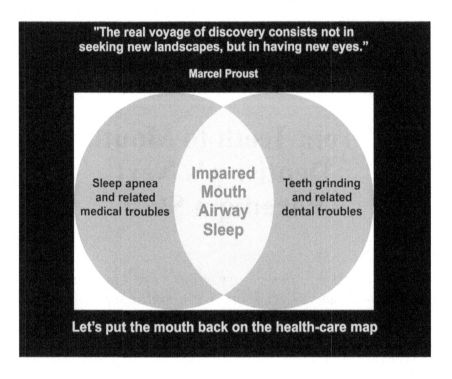

"The real voyage of discovery consists not in seeking new landscapes, but in having new eyes."

Marcel Proust

Sleep apnea and related medical troubles

Impaired Mouth Airway Sleep

Teeth grinding and related dental troubles

Let's put the mouth back on the health-care map

The solution is to make a paradigm shift—a change from one way of thinking to another.[1]

We need to move from teeth to mouth in the minds of not only patients and their doctors, dentists, and all health professionals but also employers, insurers, nonprofits, and governments at all levels.

Toward WholeHealth Integration of Mind-Body-Mouth

Fixing America's health-care costs requires identifying the root causes first. Managing the symptomatic parts have not worked, judging from America's health-care costs, as the cases of Avis, Marie, and others in this book have shown us.

Most symptoms and many diseases—heart disease, for instance—that are associated with sleep apnea ultimately have an oral origin. OSA alone is responsible for 49 percent of high-blood-pressure cases and 30 percent of heart attacks.[2] The brain needs oxygen to thrive; when it fails to get enough, health care gets costly. The Alzheimer's Association reports that Alzheimer's disease, America's sixth leading cause of death in 2013, is now "the most expensive disease in the United States." [3, 4]

A 2013 study found that "dementia represents a substantial financial burden on society, one that is similar to the financial burden of heart disease and cancer .... We found that dementia leads to total annual societal costs of $41,000 to $56,000 per case, with a total cost of $159 billion to $215 billion nationwide in 2010. Medicare paid approximately $11 billion of this cost." [5]

Such astronomical costs bind us together economically, socially, and politically. It is clearly time we start treating sources and causes. Oxygen deficiency means premature degeneration while sleep without airway obstruction is a bedrock of whole-body health. Screening for an impaired mouth and a pinched airway can only help stem the tide.

Holistic Mouth is a new solution that can resolve or reduce many sleep- and airway-related symptoms naturally at their root.

I believe that when an impaired mouth and a pinched airway are routinely included in medical, dental, and mood evaluations, health care will likely become more effective and less expensive in the long run. "Oral diseases and disorders in and of themselves affect health and well-being throughout life," states US Surgeon General Dr. David Satcher in *Oral Health in America.* [6]

As we have seen, the mouth remains left out of medical and dental care today. It is time to drop the medical/dental/mental silo mentality. Impaired Mouth is indeed that gaping "hole in the side walk" that needs patching to stop rampant Impaired Mouth Syndrome, and Holistic Mouth checkup is a start.

Educating patients on mouth-airway-sleep-wellness connections is the first step, and engaging all stakeholders in health care in a creative solution is the next step.

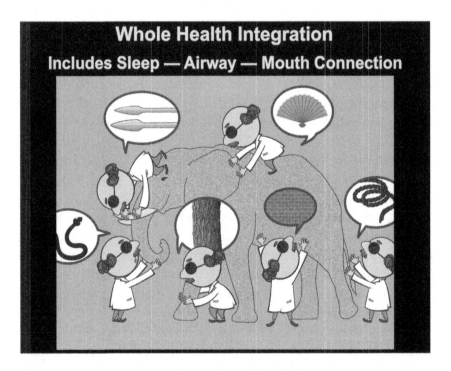

Stopping the domino effect of escalating symptoms and spiraling costs at the source requires training to help all health professionals recognize an impaired mouth as bad equipment for overall health.

Doctors focus on what they know in their areas of expertise. Dentists' eyes are used to seeing teeth, gums, and smiles. It takes additional training and much practice to see the mouth in the WholeHealth context that all parts in the body are interconnected, and that all systems are seamlessly integrated.

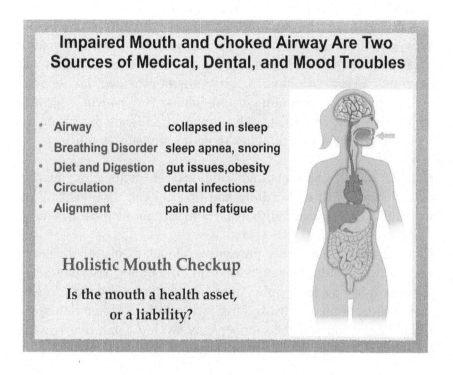

Impaired Mouth and Choked Airway Are Two Sources of Medical, Dental, and Mood Troubles

* Airway   collapsed in sleep
* Breathing Disorder   sleep apnea, snoring
* Diet and Digestion   gut issues,obesity
* Circulation   dental infections
* Alignment   pain and fatigue

Holistic Mouth Checkup

Is the mouth a health asset,
or a liability?

Dentistry's Next Paradigm Shift: From Teeth to Mouth to Integrated Well-Being

Diagnosing impaired mouths and producing Holistic Mouths across America and throughout the world are the next paradigm shift in dental care. Dentistry's history began with relief of pain and infections to fixing cavities. With the advent of the digital age, sleep medicine, and nutritional supplements, dentistry is evolving from teeth to mouth and from dental to total health and natural wellness.

In our grandparents' generation, dentures by the age of fifty were accepted without qustion. Today, parents expect their children to keep all their teeth for life. The dental profession has succeeded brilliantly in actualizing the first paradigm shift from extraction to prevention. One survey by Delta Dental found that "69 percent of Americans brush their teeth twice a day, and those who do are 22% more likely to self-report their oral health as good or better compared with those who brush less frequently."[7]

This remarkable achievement was made possible by the combination of employer-sponsored dental plans to help cover checkups and cleanings every six months, government-provided tax benefits to employers for providing health plans, and patient education by dentists and hygienists. That level of self-care is a fantastic springboard to upgrade total health with a Holistic Mouth.

Holistic Mouth checkups and solutions can predictably improve overall health just as brushing and flossing can save teeth. What would that do for your individual health and our national treasury?

Can we apply dentistry's preventive model to overall health to improve life quality and longevity? Can we copy and paste dentistry's success in saving teeth onto America's health-care system to save more hearts, brains, joints, and lives with Holistic Mouth Solutions? I believe we can and the numbers say we must, but that requires having new eyes to see the mouth's pivotal roles in total health.

Upgrade Total Health by Attending to Impaired Sleep-Airway-Mouth Connections

Shifting our focus from teeth to mouth can be powerful, benefitting individual patients, business productivity, and our national economy. But we'd have to grow new eyes to see the impaired mouth's place in our national health. This shift from teeth to mouth begins with patient education and professional recognition and training by health-care providers, and it continues with employers, health insurers, and policy makers to support the science-validated connections between oral and overall health. As US Surgeon General Dr. David Satcher states in *Oral Health America*:

The broadened meaning of oral health parallels the broadened meaning of health. In 1948 the World Health Organization expanded the definition of health to mean "a complete state of physical, mental, and social well-being, and not just the absence of infirmity." It follows that oral health must also include well-being .... We must recognize that oral health and general health are inseparable. [8]

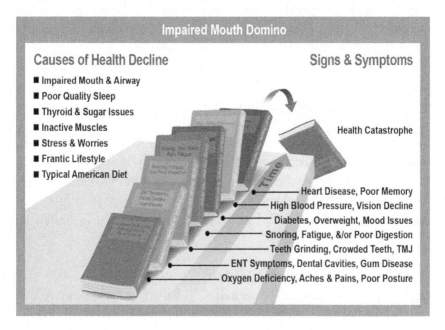

Health Insurance: Big Barrier or Beneficial Bridge?

As of this writing, there is not yet an insurance code for diagnosing an impaired mouth. There are codes for under-sized maxilla and mandible, but no benefits are quite possibly because medical and dental insurers have not yet fully understood or embraced the airway-mouth-sleep connections and its consequences. Maybe that is why the mouth is missing from nearly all the minds of doctors, dentists, insurers, and patients.

Dental insurance was instrumental to the success of preventive dentistry. But dental insurance is for tooth care, not airway obstruction, nor craniofacial orthopedic correction of impaired mouths, nor the proactive development of a Holistic Mouth for total health. Since the mouth is much more than teeth, and oral-systemic links are two-way streets, isn't it time for medical plans to cover Holistic Mouth checkupS, documentation, and treatment?

"A narrow definition of 'medically necessary dental care' currently limits oral health services for many insured persons, particularly the elderly," notes *Oral Health in America.* "You cannot be healthy without oral health. Oral health and general health should not be interpreted as separate entities. Oral health is a critical component of health and must be included in the provision of health care and the design of community programs." [9]

Insurance coverage—be it copay, deductibles, exclusions, limitations, no coverage, or other "excuses"—is the main reason that half the patients who see me do not start treating their impaired mouths and related problems. Yet to refuse coverage is to ignore all the science we have looked at—science that has clearly linked the mouth with overall health.

As US Surgeon General Dr. Richard Carmona wrote in 2003, "The report [*Oral Health in America*] ... called upon policymakers, community leaders, private industry, health professionals, the media, and the public to affirm that oral health is essential to general health and well-being and to take action. No one should suffer from oral diseases or conditions that can be effectively prevented and treated." [10]

Fourteen years later, only a medical diagnosis of obstructive sleep apnea qualifies for health insurance coverage—and only to varying degrees. This means no coverage until the patient's health has gone far enough down the hill for Obstructive Sleep Apnea to rear its ugly head—perhaps another reason for the continually rising costs of care in this country and the lack of better outcomes.

Many people still believe that if a treatment is not covered, then it is not something they need. This certainly is not the case with an impaired mouth and pinched airway. "Doctor, do you take my insurance?" is not the best question to ask for your health. Instead, it should be directed to your insurance carrier, "Why don't you cover impaired mouth diagnosis and treatment?" and to your employer, "Why do you pick such an inefficient plan for your money?"

Americans are getting fatter, losing sleep, and feeling more tired and stressed than ever. With all the brilliant minds in medicine, dentistry, insurance, and business today, surely we can find ways to deliver a Holistic Mouth to many more Americans to improve sleep, raise productivity, and reduce disease care cost.

It is time for employers to provide better coverage options for their employees, and it's time for health insurers to step up and create more effective plans that say YES to better total health by mouth. It's time to cover the diagnosis and treatment of an impaired mouth, just like six-month dental checkups and cleanings. Recognizing Impaired Mouth Syndrome and providing coverage for Holistic Mouth solutions can help reverse or mitigate this costly Impaired Mouth domino.

Healthier Outcomes Require Upgraded Strategies and Tactics

An impaired mouth is a slow kill. A Holistic Mouth is a fast heal. So what actions are needed to actualize Holistic Mouth as a solution?

Employers and insurers need to see that paying for Holistic Mouth checkups and solutions is good business. Eliminating the mouth as a source of chronic pain, obstructive sleep apnea, and teeth grinding can greatly reduce downstream costs while raising health and upgrading life quality.

Better media coverage can help drive better insurance coverage. The number of people suffering from an undiagnosed impaired mouth and related sleep troubles, chronic pain, fatigue, snoring, sleep apnea, and teeth grinding is enormous, and the cost of managing their complications is bankrupting people and nations.

For public health officials and policy planners, a dental visit can be a useful opportunity to screen for oral-systemic issues and to refer patients for early medical testing and intervention. "In many cases," notes Delta Dental, "a dentist may be the first health care provider to diagnose a health problem in its early stages since many people have regular oral examinations and see their dentist more often than their physician." [11]

Dental offices certified to provide Holistic Mouth checkups can be valuable resources already in place to reduce medical costs and morbidity related to chronic pain and sleep apnea. Until health insurers and employers see the light, what can patients do, and how can their doctors help?

All Health-Caring Professionals Can Help

Every health professional who care about patient's well-being can help put the mouth and airway back on the body map by recognizing an impaired mouth's signs and symptoms. By attending an online webinar, non-dental health professionals can become Impaired Mouth Investigators. By participating in a one-day seminar, they can become Holistic Mouth Consultants with the ability and opportunity to integrate a systemically-sound mouth program into their patient care."

Patients know intuitively that all parts of the body are interconnected, and they appreciate health professionals who know how to integrate mind-body-mouth.

Trained as doctors of the Holistic Mouth, dentists are in a strategic position to recognize orofacial signs of medical problems and the systemic consequences of an impaired mouth on the airway, blood pressure, sleep, and memory early on. Considerable training beyond dental school and teeth-centered seminars are needed for dentists to acquire the eyes, knowledge, and skill set of a mouth doctor to diagnose and re-engineer an impaired mouth.

Patients: How to Take Charge of Your Health by Taking Charge of Your Mouth

For the patient's part, you need to know if you have an impaired mouth as an overlooked health liability. Getting a Holistic Mouth checkup by a trained Holistic Mouth doctor is the first step. Insurance coverage varies from surprisingly good to nothing, and you can expect denial, long holds on the phone, and jumping through insurance-plan hoops, based on my patients' experience. The time is ripe for health-insurance innovations from product design to claims review to customer service.

Until then, you can expect to pay out of pocket for Holistic Mouth checkups and impaired mouth treatment, depending on your plan level being platinum, gold, silver, bronze, or hot air. To get more coverage, you will need to take steps to advocate for yourself through pressure on employers to select more integrative health plans and pressure on elected officials charged with healthcare policy and related spending.

I propose that a Holistic Mouth be recognized as an essential prerequisite for building and maintaining total health. I will devote my life energy to the cause of making Holistic Mouth happen for as many people as possible through patient education, professional training, Holistic Mouth doctor certification, and integrative collaboration among all health professionals to include this strategy as a natural solution to reduce pain and fatigue and to improve sleep and energy.

With the right diagnosis of the missing pieces in America's health-care system and with a concerted effort to implement the treatment plan needed to fix our disease care costs, we can improve oral-systemic health and decrease health-care costs.

Holistic Mouth Bites

- An impaired mouth is a slow kill. A Holistic Mouth is a fast heal. Holistic Mouth as a solution can predictably improve overall health just as brushing and flossing has done for dental health.

- Recognizing and treating an impaired mouth and a pinched airway early on can help save a brain, a heart, many teeth, and much more down the road. Diagnosing impaired mouth and producing Holistic Mouth across America and around the world is the next paradigm shift in dental care.

- It's time to provide for insurance coverage for the diagnosis and treatment of impaired mouth, just like six-month dental checkups and cleanings.

Epilogue

A Better Second Half of Life: A Chair-Side Chat

80% of all chronic pain and illness originate between the scalp and the clavicle.

– Dietrich Klinghardt, MD, PhD

"Why are so many teeth falling apart on me all of a sudden?" Suzette asked when she came into my office for a broken filling. "I had a bunch of cavities filled as a teenager," continued this forty-eight-year-old mom of two teens, "but not much has happened since until these two broken teeth and that abscess."

"Chalk it up to mileage and excessive wear and tear," I explained. "It's like driving the best car with the front end out of alignment. Your broken and sensitive teeth may well have to do with the combination of old fillings leaking at the seams and causing cavities, AND the stress of jaw clenching and teeth grinding."

"Nothing personal, but I get super anxious whenever I have to go to the dentist." At fifty pounds overweight, Suzette works hard to make ends meet but admits to feeling tired. "Oh, how I wish for a trouble-free mouth for the second half of my life!"

"It's still within your reach—when you begin to address the causes of your daily and nightly stress."

"I know all about your theory of the six-foot tiger in a three-foot cage, but I just don't have the money to fix mine right now."

"There's a right time for everything. At this time, you have a couple dental fires to put out," I answered. "If you really want a better second half of life, though, we can revisit the consequences of ignoring your oral contributions to your total health at your next checkup and cleaning visit."

"I'd like that, yes."

Every dental visit is an opportunity to connect the mouth with its owner and his or her total health.

Oral Airway Contributions to Total Health

In its simplest sense, "WholeHealth" means that all parts of the body are interconnected. Gum inflammation, for instance, has been linked to Alzheimer's, heart disease, cancer, and more. We might even say that every disease, pain, and illness has an oral connection until proven otherwise.

Suzette's dental troubles do not exist by themselves, as if her teeth were not a part of her body. Instead, dental troubles are bodily reactions to some persistent stress, be it mental-emotional, nutritional, or habitual jaw clenching and teeth grinding. Whatever the stress, it knocks the body's ability to run itself off balance.

When teeth are stressed, so is the whole body. Book 2 of this *Holistic Mouth Solutions* series covers more ripple effects of living and sleeping with a pinched airway inside an impaired mouth beyond sleep apnea, including why teeth grinding happens and how it ruins more than teeth. We will explore the relationships between stress, being overweight, chronic fatigue, and an impaired mouth. We will look at the evidence linking diabetes and other leading chronic diseases with the six-foot tiger in a three-foot cage.

And we will go deeper into what you can do about it, taking charge of your own health and well-being, creating the healthy, happy life you desire.

Need More Information?

Many more resources are available for you at HolisticMouthSolutions. com, including:

- Referrals for Holistic Mouth doctors and more resources

- Further educational opportunities such as webinars and resources for patients

- Information for dentists aspiring to become certified Holistic Mouth doctors

- Information for non-dental health professionals to become Impaired Mouth Investigators and Holistic Mouth Consultants

- Information for businesses or organizations seeking Dr. Liao as a speaker or consultant

Got an Impaired Mouth? Discover Your Holistic Mouth Score

Is your mouth helping or hurting your health? Is your mouth an asset to your sleep and energy, or a liability? This can be a life-changing question. Discovering your Holistic Mouth score is the place to start finding some answers.

This self-survey begins to illuminate your mouth's structural contributions to medical, dental, and mental-emotional symptoms. It's essentially a checklist of the more common orofacial, dental, and bodily signs and symptoms of an impaired mouth.

The higher your score, the more likely you have been living with an impaired mouth for a long time.

You can access and download the digital versions of the following templates and materials at: http://holisticmouthsolutions.com/

Holistic Mouth Score

Mouth	Score	Body	Score
Snoring, morning dry mouth	0 1	Gasping or choking in sleep	0 1
Teeth grinding, jaw	0 1	Neck, shoulder, or back pain; headaches	0 1
Mouth breathing, chapped lips	0 1	Erectile dysfunction or PMS	0 1
Persistent/wandering dental sensitivity	0 1	High blood pressure, heart disease	0 1
Gum recession and/or redness	0 1	Diabetes type 2, bloating after meals	0 1
Clicking/locking jaw joints, zigzag jaw opening	0 1	Weight gain, pot belly; acid reflux	0 1
Morning headache and/or sore jaws	0 1	Daytime sleepiness, fatigue	0 1
Deep overbite or underbite (weak chin)	0 1	Senile memory, ADD/ADHD	0 1
Frequent cavities or broken/chipped teeth	0 1	Frequent colds, flu, and skin disorders	0 1
Teeth prints on the sides of the tongue	0 1	Obstructive sleep apnea from a sleep test	0 1
Bony outgrowth on palate or inside lower jaw	0 1	Stuffy/runny nose, scratchy/itchy throat	0 1
Sunken lips and reverse smile curve (sad)	0 1	Forward head: ears ahead of shoulders	0 1
History of teeth extractions for braces	0 1	Waking up to urinate more than once	0 1
Bulge under lower jaw, double chin	0 1	Large neck size (M>17, W>15)	0 1
History of lots of dental work + medical symptoms	0 1	Poor digestion and elimination	0 1
Malocclusion (crowded teeth)	0 1	Depression, anxiety, grouchiness	0 1

Please note that the Holistic Mouth score is not, at this time, a diagnostic tool. No study has been done on it. But it is an excellent conversation starter with your doctor or dentist to rule out an impaired mouth. This is how I encourage you to use it—to get the ball rolling so that you can get on the path to improved health and vitality.

Holistic Mouth Checkup

The next step is a Holistic Mouth checkup by a trained health professional, including appropriate imaging of the jaws and oral airway, as well as a sleep test (as needed) to confirm an impaired mouth diagnosis.

A dental checkup covers the teeth and gums, which is an important foundation, of course. A Holistic Mouth checkup builds on that foundation by examining the mouth's role in whole-body health through ABCDES: alignment, breathing, circulation, digestion, energy, and sleep.

To find a properly trained Holistic Mouth doctor near you who can provide you with a Holistic Mouth checkup, visit HolisticMouthSolutions.com. Because Holistic Mouth is a brand new concept and practice, Holistic Mouth doctors will be in very short supply. If you cannot find one, please consider referring your own dentist to this website.

Your Daytime Sleepiness:
The Epworth Sleepiness Scale

The Epworth sleepiness scale is a tool doctors use to evaluate daytime sleepiness—one of the most common signs of sleep apnea and often a clue to airway issues that result from an impaired mouth.

Think about each of the situations listed below, and then rate how likely you are to doze off while engaged in the activities described:

0 = not at all likely
1 = slightly likely
2 = moderately likely
3 = very likely

Situation	Chance of dozing
Sitting and reading	
Watching TV	
Sitting in a public place	
Riding as a passenger in a car for one hour	
Lying down in the afternoon	
Sitting and talking with someone	
Sitting quietly after a lunch with no alcohol	
Stopped for a few minutes in traffic	

Source: The Epworth Sleepiness Scale, by Dr. Murray Johns,
http://epworthsleepinessscale.com/about-the-ess/

The average score is four to eight. If you score higher than this, you should talk with your doctor—especially if your score is sixteen or above.

Please note that the survey presented here is not the official diagnostic tool but is shared as a means of self-assessment, to recognize whether daytime sleepiness is an issue for you so that you can seek help as needed from your health-care providers.

Children's Holistic Mouth Development: A Parents' Guide

Your child's orofacial and dental development starts well before birth. In the WholeHealth approach, a partnership between parents and a doctor of Holistic Mouth is encouraged, with the following ideals in mind:

Preconception

- Sound and sensible nutrition for six to twelve months

- A dental checkup to ensure healthy teeth and sound gums for the mom-to-be

- A Holistic Mouth checkup to rule out a pinched airway and more

Immediately after Birth

- Breast-feeding – nature's way for a baby to develop a wide upper jaw

- Check for tongue-tie and upper lip-tie if breast latch is problematic.

- Check for cranial distortion from birth trauma, and seek a cranial osteopathic doctor or craniosacral therapist if crying, irritability, colic, and/or spit-up persist

First Eighteen Months

- After about a year of breast-feeding, follow Baby-Led Weaning: http://www.babyledweaning.com/.

- During weaning, watch for signs of allergies, ear infections, stuffy nose, mouth breathing, and dry lips.

- For nutritional information to grow good teeth and faces, visit the Weston A. Price Foundation: http://www.wapf.org.

- Once your child can walk and run, watch for a slouched posture with forward head, and encourage active play using all four limbs rather than just the two thumbs.

Dental Care and Holistic Mouth Checkups

- Brush teeth as soon as they come into mouth to develop this healthy habit.

- Take your child to a family or pediatric dentist once their molars start to come in.

- A positive first impression can last a lifetime. A helpful way to visit the dentist for the first time is as a guest during a parent's or older sibling's checkup/cleaning.

- Parents are responsible for children's teeth brushing and flossing until nine or ten years old.

- Space between front teeth is desirable in baby teeth, except in cases of tongue thrust or lip-tie.

- Look for facial symmetry, and watch for the red flags listed below.

Red Flags
in Children's Dental-Facial Development

- Tongue-tie or tongue thrust
- No lip seal; uneven eyes
- Narrow / uneven nostrils
- Chapped lips, weak chin
- Ear-nose-throat infections
- Teeth grinding, snoring
- Finger-sucking, bed-wetting
- Tired or hyperactive

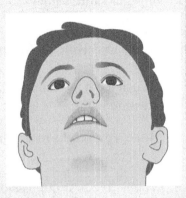

*Have the child tip her/his head back and the
parent can look up from below the chin*

Red Flags of Impaired Mouth
Development in Children

Medical Clues

_____Allergies, frequent colds, inflamed tonsils, headaches

_____Earaches, recurrent ear infections, or stuffiness

_____Accidents, head trauma, broken nose, falls, scars from stitches

_____Attention deficit or hyperactivity

_____Tiredness, low energy, socially withdrawn

254

Facial Appearance

_____Forward head (ear hole ahead of shoulder point in profile),
slumped posture

_____Uneven ears or eyes

_____Narrow nostrils

_____Small (weak) chin

_____Dry or parched lips, lack of lip seal

_____Deep chin cleft

_____"Gummy" smile

_____Overly long "horse" face or overly flat "bulldog" midface

Dental Clues

_____Teeth grinding

_____Thumb-sucking

_____Open bite (space between upper and lower front teeth for
thumb or tongue)

_____Crowded or crooked (rotated or turned) front teeth

_____Deep bite (upper front teeth overlap more than half of lower
front teeth)

_____Crossbite (any lower front or back tooth/teeth)

_____Mismatched upper and lower dental midlines

_____Jaw opening-closing zigzagging or deviated instead of
straight/smooth

Lifelong Benefits of an Early Holistic Mouth Checkup

I recommend a Holistic Mouth checkup for the mother-to-be long
before conception. For the newborn, tongue-tie should be evaluated
right after birth if there is any breast-feeding difficulty.

Holistic Mouth checkup starts the first time a child sees a dentist trained as a Holistic Mouth doctor who will check all the signs and symptoms of impaired mouth—no later than age two—and every six months thereafter.

Holistic Mouth checkups, in collaboration with integrative health professionals and consistent with WholeHealth principles, can help facilitate the development of a Holistic Mouth to grow children into fully potentiated adults. The benefits of a Holistic Mouth can include:

- Avoiding extraction of permanent teeth or jaw surgery in many cases

- Growing into full potential academically, athletically, and socially

- Mitigation of risks for snoring, sleep apnea, teeth grinding, chronic pain and fatigue, and more

- Living a healthy, enjoyable life with far fewer health complications

- Feeling and looking like a winner!

The age of seven or eight is a good time for a full evaluation, including preferably a 3D-CT scan and cephalometric analysis of the craniofacial skeleton. This allows for early correction of habitual mouth breathing, tongue-tie, and/or orthopedic misalignment or under/over-development while the bones are still soft and flexible.

Acknowledgments and Gratitude

This book is the fruit of too many people to name here. I am grateful to all the patients who have contributed to this book with their stories and images, and to all other patients who have added to my experience through the years.

I am grateful, too, to all the instructors who have taught me—from dental school to postgraduate seminars in dentistry, medicine, and integrative health, as well as those who have contributed to this book. You know who you are.

I thank all my friends and colleagues who have encouraged and supported me through the years of writing this book: Jasmine Ma, Dr. Sharon Fan, Dr. Brendan Stack, Dr. Jay Gerber, Dr. Richard Beistle, Dr. Dennis Bailey, Dr. G. Dave Singh, Dr. Louisa Williams, Dr. George Yu, Dr. Robert Walker, Dr. Je-yang Jau and his graphic artist Jia-jun Tsai in Taiwan, Demerie Faitler, Lisa Verigin, Ken Sandler, Sue Glass, Gwen Hernandez, Jessie Martin, David Gruder, Linda Kaye, my office staff, my brother Allen, Aunt Grace Lin, and publisher Robbin Simons and her superb team at Crescendo Publishing.

About the Author

Dr. Liao is a holistic dentist and mouth doctor devoted to helping patients turn back illness and turn on wellness with Holistic Mouth Solutions. He blends leading edge technology with old-fashioned TLC for children and adults at WholeHealth Dental Center in Falls Church, Virginia.

Dr. Liao's professional mission is to help build whole body health with a holistic mouth — one that is an asset to whole body health rather than a liability. Since dental school, Dr. Liao has been interested in teeth grinding: "Why would the body mutilate the hardest tissue it has?!" Holistic Mouth Solutions result from Dr. Liao's pursuit to find the root cause of teeth grinding and better overall health by mouth.

For patients wishing to cultivate a more holistic mouth style to support overall health, Dr. Liao teaches WholeHealth Wellness Seminars. Dr. Liao also offers Holistic Mouth Seminars to help aspiring dentists and all health professionals to become certified holistic mouth doctors. More information at HolisticMouthSolutions.com.

Dr. Liao is a U.S. citizen born and raised in Taiwan until age 16. He graduated from Brown University with an engineering degree, and Doctor of Dental Surgery from Case School of Dental Medicine. Since dental school, he has taken extensive post-graduate training in integrative medicine, oral-systemic dentistry, nutrition, cranial osteopathy, chiropractics, nutrition, and studies in Traditional Chinese Medicine.

He is a board-certified general dentist with Masterships in both the Academy of General Dentistry and the International Academy of Biological Dentistry and Medicine (IABDM). He is the current president of IABDM.

Dr. Liao has been a speaker at the International College of Integrative Medicine, Weston A. Price Foundation, the Holistic Moms' Network, Take Back Your Health Conference, Academy of Integrative Health and Medicine, and International Academy of Biological Dentistry and Medicine, among others.

Dr. Liao's personal interests includes classical music, organic lifestyle, science, world cuisine and culture, learning and teaching health-building skills, and research connecting cranial-facial-dental development with nutrition and lifestyle habits.

Connect with the Author

Dr. Felix Liao, DDS, MAGD, ABGD, MIABDM

Address: P.O. Box 3325, Merrifield, Virginia 22116
Phone: 703-385-6425

Websites: www.HolisticMouthSolutions.com
www.WholeHealthDentalCenter.com

Email: DrFelix@HolisticMouthSolutions.com

Facebook: https://www.facebook.com/HolisticMouthSolutions

LinkedIn: https://www.linkedin.com/company/HolisticMouthSolutions

Twitter: www.twitter.com/DrFelixLiao

Instagram: HolisticMouthSolutions

References

Introduction

1. U.S. Department of Health and Human Services, "Chapter 2: The Craniofacial Complex," in Oral Health in America: A Report of the Surgeon General (Rockville, MD: U.S. Department of Health and Human Services, National Institute of Dental and Craniofacial Research, National Institutes of Health, 2000)

Ch. 1 Redeveloping Impaired Mouth Benefits the Whole Body: The Case of Smithy

1. Murray W. Johns, "1997 Version of ESS," The Epworth Sleepiness Scale, http://epworthsleepinessscale.com/1997-version-ess/.

Ch. 2 Good Mouth Bad Mouth

1. U.S. Department of Health and Human Services, *Oral Health in America: A Report of the Surgeon General* (Rockville, MD: U.S. Department of Health and Human Services, National Institute of Dental and Craniofacial Research, National Institutes of Health, 2000), 10–11, http://www.nidcr.nih.gov/DataStatistics/SurgeonGeneral/sgr/welcome.htm.

2. Etsuko Miyao and others, "The Role of Malocclusion in Non-obese Patients with Obstructive Sleep Apnea Syndrome," *Internal Medicine* 47, no. 18 (2008): 1573–

1578, DOI: 10.2169/internalmedicine.47.0717, PMID: 18797115.

Ch. 3: Your Mouth-Body Connections

1. Ide M, Harris M, Stevens A, Sussams R, Hopkins V, Culliford D, et al. (2016) Periodontitis and Cognitive Decline in Alzheimer's Disease. PLoS ONE 11(3): e0151081. doi:10.1371/journal.pone.0151081

2. Bradley Bale and Amy Doneen, "Guarantee for Arterial Wellness: Medical-Dental Collaboration Is Critical" (lecture, International Academy of Biological Dentistry and Medicine Annual Meeting, October, 2013).

3. Bradley Bale and Amy Doneen, "Chapter 3: Red Flags — Are You at Risk?" in Beat The Heart Attack Gene: The Revolutionary Plan to Prevent Heart Disease, Stroke, and Diabetes (Nashville, TN: Turner Publishing Company, 2014), 43–44.

4. Tanja Pessi and others, "Bacterial Signatures in Thrombus Aspirates of Patients with Myocardial Infarction," *Circulation* 127 (2013): 1219–1228, DOI: 10.1161/CIRCULATIONAHA.112.001254, PMID: 23418311.

5. Mikko J. Pyysalo and others, "The Connection Between Ruptured Cerebral Aneurysms and Odontogenic Bacteria," *Journal of Neurology, Neurosurgery, and Psychiatry* 84, no. 11 (2013): 1214 –1218, DOI: 10.1136/jnnp-2012-304635.

6. Seymour M. Antelman and others, "Tail Pinch-Induced Eating, Gnawing, and Licking Behavior in Rats: Dependence on Nigrostriatal Dopamine System," *Brain Research* 99, no. 2 (1975): 319–337, DOI: 10.1016/0006-8993(75)90032-3, PMID: 1182545.

7. Kristine Yaffe and others, "Sleep-Disordered Breathing, Hypoxia, and Risk of Mild Cognitive Impairment and Dementia in Older Women," *Journal of the American Medical Association* 306, no. 6 (2011): 613–619, DOI: 10.1001/jama.2011.1115, PMID: 21828324.

8. Kiran Devulapally, Raymond Pongonis Jr., and Rami Khayat, "OSA: The New Cardiovascular Disease, Part II: Overview of Cardiovascular Diseases Associated with Obstructive Sleep Apnea," *Heart Failure Reviews* 14, no. 3 (2009): 155–164, DOI: 10.1007/s10741-008-9101-2, PMID: 18758946.

9. Richard H. Nagelberg, DDS, "The Oral-Systemic Connection," *Dental Economics* 101, no. 6, http://www.dentaleconomics.com/articles/print/volume-101/issue-6/practice/the-oral-systemic-connection.html.

10. Dr. Joseph Mercola, "The Greatest Nutrition Researcher of the 20th Century," Mercola.com, Oct. 6, 2007, http://articles.mercola.com/sites/articles/archive/2007/10/06/the-greatest-nutrition-researcher-of-the-twentieth-century.aspx.

11. Jerry Tennant, MD, "Master's Class, Tennant BioModulator, Mind-Body Connection" (lecture, Dallas, TX, Feb. 21–22, 2014).

12. Louisa Williams, email message to author, June 22, 2015.

13. Reyes Enciso and others, "Comparison of Cone-Beam CT Parameters and Sleep Questionnaires in Sleep Apnea Patients and Control Subjects," Oral Surgery, Oral Medicine, Oral Pathology, Oral Radiology, and Endodontology 109, no. 2 (2010): 285–293, DOI: 10.1016/j.tripleo.2009.09.033, PMID: 20123412.

Ch. 4: Saving His Life & Her Sanity

1. U.S. Department of Health and Human Services, "Chapter 2: The Craniofacial Complex," in *Oral Health in America: A Report of the Surgeon General* (Rockville, MD: U.S. Department of Health and Human Services, National Institute of Dental and Craniofacial Research, National Institutes of Health, 2000)

2. Yu-Shu Huang and others, "Short Lingual Frenulum and Obstructive Sleep Apnea in Children," *International Journal of Pediatric Research* 1, no. 1 (2015), http://clinmedjournals.org/articles/ijpr/ijpr-1-003.pdf.

3. Reyes Enciso and others, "Comparison of Cone-Beam CT Parameters and Sleep Questionnaires in Sleep Apnea Patients and Control Subjects," Oral Surgery, Oral Medicine, Oral Pathology, Oral Radiology, and Endodontology 109, no. 2 (2010): 285–293, DOI: 10.1016/j.tripleo.2009.09.033, PMID: 20123412.

4. "Obstructive Sleep Apnea" (Darien, IL: American Academy of Sleep Medicine, 2008), http://www.aasmnet.org/resources/factsheets/sleepapnea.pdf.

5. Puneet S. Garcha, Loutfi S. Aboussouan, and Omar Minai, "Sleep-Disordered Breathing," in Disease Management, an online medical reference (Lyndhurst, OH: Cleveland Clinic, 2000–2015), http://www.clevelandclinicmeded.com/medicalpubs/diseasemanagement/pulmonary/sleep-disordered-breathing/.

Ch. 5: CSI for Your Mouth

1. Thomas S. Kuhn, "The Structure of Scientific Revolutions", p. 67, Second Edition, Enlarged, The University of Chicago Press, Chicago, 1970 (1962)

2. Xavier Barceló and others, "Oropharyngeal Examination to Predict Sleep Apnea Severity," *Archives of Otolaryngology — Head & Neck Surgery* 137, no. 10 (2011): 990–996, DOI: 10.1001/archoto.2011.176, PMID: 22006776.

3. Etsuko Myiao and others, "The Role of Malocclusion in Non-obese Patients with Obstructive Sleep Apnea Syndrome," *Internal Medicine* 47, no. 18 (2008): 1573–1578, DOI: 10.2169/internalmedicine.47.0717, PMID: 18797115.

4. William C. Lee and W. Stephan Eakle, "Possible Role of Tensile Stress in the Etiology of Cervical Erosive Lesions of Teeth," *Journal of Prosthetic Dentistry* 52, no. 3 (1984): 374–380, DOI: 10.1016/0022-3913(84)90448-7, PMID: 6592336.

5. J.S. Rees, "The Effect of Variation in Occlusal Loading on the Development of Abfraction Lesions: A Finite Element Study," Journal of Oral Rehabilitation 29, no. 2 (2002): 188–193, DOI: 10.1046/j.1365-2842.2002.00836.x, http://www.fo.ufu.br/sites/fo.ufu.br/files/Anexos/Comunicados/Rees_JS_2002.pdf.

6. G. Dave Singh, "Guest Editorial on the Etiology and Significance of Palatal and Mandibular Tori," CRANIO: The Journal of Craniomandibular & Sleep Practice 28, no. 4 (2010): 213–215, PMID: 21032973, http://www.smileprofessionals.com/uploads/Cranio-2010-Tori-Singh.pdf.

Ch. 6: Damaging Domino Effects of Impaired Mouth

7. G. Dave Singh and James A. Krumholtz, Epigenetic Orthodontics in Adults (Chatsworth, CA: Smile Foundation, 2009).

8. Shiroh Isono and others, "Anatomy of Pharynx in Patients with Obstructive Sleep Apnea and in Normal Subjects," *Journal of Applied Physiology* 82, no. 4 (1997): 1319–1326, http://jap.physiology.org/content/82/4/1319, PMID: 9104871.

9. Sonal B. Dudhia and Bhavin B. Dudhia, "Undetected Hypothyroidism: A Rare Dental Diagnosis," *Journal of Oral and Maxillofacial Pathology* 18, no. 2 (2014): 315–319, DOI: 10.4103/0973-029X.140922, PMID: 25328321.

10. Mark Starr, Hypothyroidism Type 2: The Epidemic (Columbia, MO: Mark Starr Trust, 2011), 119.

11. Roseane C. Marchiori and others, "Improvement of Blood Inflammatory Marker Levels in Patients with Hypothyroidism Under Levothyroxine Treatment," *BMC Endocrine Disorders* 15, no. 32 (2015), DOI: 10.1186/s12902-015-0032-3, PMID: 26100072.

Ch. 7: A Deeper Look at Obstructive Sleep Apnea

1. William C. Dement and Merrill M. Mitler, "It's Time to Wake Up to the Importance of Sleep Disorders," *Journal of the American Medical Association* 269, no. 12 (1993): 1548–1550, DOI: 10.1001/jama.1993.03500120086032, PMID: 8445820.

2. Vishesh Kapur and others, "The Medical Cost of Undiagnosed Sleep Apnea," *SLEEP* 22, no. 6 (1999):

749–755, http://www.journalsleep.org/ViewAbstract. aspx?pid=24161, PMID: 10505820.

3. "Obstructive Sleep Apnea" (Darien, IL: American Academy of Sleep Medicine, 2008), http://www.aasmnet.org/ resources/factsheets/sleepapnea.pdf.

4. "Obstructive Sleep Apnea" (Darien, IL: American Academy of Sleep Medicine, 2008), http://www.aasmnet.org/ resources/factsheets/sleepapnea.pdf.

5. Atul Malhotra and David P. White, "Obstructive Sleep Apnea," *Lancet* 360, no. 9328 (2002): 237–245, DOI: 10.1016/   S0140-6736(02)09464-310.1016/S0140-6736(02)09464-3.

6. Terry Young and others, "The Occurrence of Sleep-Disordered Breathing Among Middle-Aged Adults," *New England Journal of Medicine* 328, no. 17 (1993): 1230–235, DOI: 10.1056/NEJM199304293281704, PMID: 8464434.

7. Terry Young and others, "Sleep-Disordered Breathing and Mortality: Eighteen-Year Follow-up of the Wisconsin Sleep Cohort," *SLEEP* 31, no. 8 (2008): 1071–1078, http://www. journalsleep.org/ViewAbstract.aspx?pid=27213, PMID: 18714778.

8. Andrew Schriber, "Obstructive Sleep Apnea – Adults," MedlinePlus, https://www.nlm.nih.gov/medlineplus/ency/ article/000811.htm.

Ch. 8: Resolving High Blood Pressure Without Medication

1. Jo-Dee L. Lattimore, David S. Celermajer, and Ian Wilcox, "Obstructive Sleep Apnea and Cardiovascular Disease,"

Journal of the American College of Cardiology 41, no. 9 (2003): 1429–1437, DOI: 10.1016/S0735-1097(03)00184-0, PMID: 12742277.

2. "Understanding Blood Pressure Readings," American Heart Association, http://www.heart.org/HEARTORG/Conditions/HighBloodPressure/AboutHighBloodPressure/Understanding-Blood-Pressure-Readings_UCM_301764_Article.jsp.

3. Kazuya Yoshida, "Effect on Blood Pressure of Oral Appliance Therapy for Sleep Apnea Syndrome," *International Journal of Prosthodontics* 19, no.1 (2006): 61–66, http://www.quintpub.com/journals/ijp/abstract.php?iss2_id=184&article_id=2102&article=17&title=Effect - .VhgFWyjZg07, PMID: 16479762.

Ch. 9: Sleep Apnea Solution: CPAP Dependence or Oral Appliance Development?

1. "Obstructive Sleep Apnea" (Darien, IL: American Academy of Sleep Medicine, 2008), http://www.aasmnet.org/resources/factsheets/sleepapnea.pdf.

2. See Note 1.

3. Clete A. Kushida and others, "Practice Parameters for the Treatment of Snoring and Obstructive Sleep Apnea with Oral Appliances: An Update for 2005; An American Academy of Sleep Medicine Report," *SLEEP* 29, no. 2 (2006): 240–243, PMID: 16494092, http://www.aasmnet.org/resources/practiceparameters/pp_update_oralapplicance.pdf.

4. Kannan Ramar and others, "Clinical Practice Guideline for the Treatment of Obstructive Sleep Apnea and Snoring with Oral Appliance Therapy: An Update for 2015," *Journal of Clinical Sleep Medicine* 11, no. 7 (2015): 773–827, DOI: 10.5664/jcsm.4858, http://www.aasmnet.org/Resources/clinicalguidelines/Oral_appliance-OSA.pdf.

5. Canadian Agency for Drugs and Technologies in Health, "Oral Appliances for Treatment of Snoring and Obstructive Sleep Apnea: A Review of Clinical Effectiveness" *CADTH Technology Overviews* 1, no. 1 (2010): e0107, http://www.ncbi.nlm.nih.gov/pmc/articles/PMC3411138/.

6. Andrew S.L. Chan, Robert W.W. Lee, and Peter A. Cistulli, "Dental Appliance Treatment for Obstructive Sleep Apnea," *Chest* 132, no. 2 (2007): 693–699, DOI: 10.1378/chest.06-2038, PMID: 17699143.

7. Glenn T. Clark and others, "A Crossover Study Comparing the Efficacy of Continuous Positive Airway Pressure with Anterior Mandibular Positioning Devices on Patients with Obstructive Sleep Apnea," *Chest* 109, no. 6 (1996): 1477–1483, DOI: 10.1378/chest.109.6.1477, PMID: 8769497.

8. Kathleen A. Ferguson and others, "A Randomized Crossover Study of an Oral Appliance Vs Nasal-Continuous Positive Airway Pressure in the Treatment of Mild-Moderate Obstructive Sleep Apnea," *Chest* 109, no. 5 (1996): 1269–1275, DOI: 10.1378/chest.109.5.1269, PMID: 8625679.

9. Helen Gotsopoulos, John J. Kelly, and Peter A. Cistulli, "Oral Appliance Therapy Reduces Blood Pressure in Obstructive Sleep Apnea: A Randomized, Controlled Trial," *SLEEP* 27, no. 5 (2004): 934–941, http://journalsleep.org/ViewAbstract.aspx?pid=26027, PMID: 15453552.

10. Kathleen A. Ferguson and others, "Oral Appliances for Snoring and Obstructive Sleep Apnea: A Review," *SLEEP* 29, no. 2 (2006): 244–262, http://www.journalsleep.org/ViewAbstract.aspx?pid=26465, PMID: 16494093.

11. Bing Lam and others, "Randomised Study of Three Non-surgical Treatments in Mild to Moderate Obstructive Sleep Apnoea," *Thorax* 62, no. 4 (2007): 354–359, DOI: 10.1136/thx.2006.063644, PMID: 17121868.

12. Hiroko Tsuda and others, "Craniofacial Changes After Two Years of Nasal Continuous Positive Airway Pressure Use in Patients with Obstructive Sleep Apnea," *Chest* 138, no. 4 (2010): 870–874, DOI: 10.1378/chest.10-0678, PMID: 20616213.

Ch. 10: The Rarely Addressed Game Changer: The Maxilla

1. Donald H. Enlow, Robert E. Moyers, and William W. Merow, Handbook of Facial Growth (Philadelphia: W.B. Saunders Co., 1975).

2. Weston A. Price, Nutrition and Physical Degeneration (Lemon Grove, CA: Price-Pottenger Nutrition Foundation, 2008). An earlier version of the book can be read at http://gutenberg.net.au/ebooks02/0200251h.html or http://journeytoforever.org/farm_library/price/pricetoc.html.

3. Francis M. Pottenger Jr., Pottenger's Cats: A Study in Nutrition, 2nd ed. (Lemon Grove, CA: Price-Pottenger Nutrition Foundation, 1995).

4. Sally Fallon, *Nourishing Traditions Diet*, New Trends Publishing (2003) 2nd ed.

Ch. 12: Better Sleep, Better Health, Better Looks: The Maxilla Triple Win

1. Yu-shu Huang, Stacey Quo, Andrew Berkowski, Christian Guilleminault, Short Lingual Frenulum and Obstructive Sleep Apnea in Children. International Journal of Pediatric Research 2015, 1:003.

2. Ranji Varghese, Nathan G. Adams, Nancy L. Slocumb, Christopher F. Viozzi, Kannan Ramar, and Eric J. Olson. Maxillomandibular Advancement in the Management of Obstructive Sleep Apnea. International Journal of Otolaryngology, Volume 2012 (2012), Article ID 373025, 8 pages: http://dx.doi.org/10.1155/2012/373025

3. James A. McNamara Jr., Components of Class II Malocclusion in Children 8–10 Years of Age. The Angle Orthodontist: July 1981, Vol. 51, No. 3, pp. 177-202, Figures 6 and 7.

4. G. Dave Singh and James A. Krumholtz, *Epigenetic Orthodontics in Adults* (Chatsworth, CA: Smile Foundation, 2009), page 27.

5. G. Dave Singh and James A. Krumholtz, *Epigenetic Orthodontics in Adults* (Chatsworth, CA: Smile Foundation, 2009), page 27.

6. Baccetti T, McGill JS, Franchi L, McNamara JA, Jr, Tollaro I. Skeletal effects of early treatment of Class III malocclusion with maxillary expansion and face-mask therapy Am J Orthod Dentofacial Orthop.1998;113:333-43.

7. Aelred C. Fonder, "Dental Distress Syndrome Quantified," *Basal Facts* 9, no. 4 (1987): 141–167, http://www. betterhealththruresearch.com/OldSite/DDS.pdf.

8. Etsuko Miyao and others, "The Role of Malocclusion in Non-obese Patients with Obstructive Sleep Apnea Syndrome," *Internal Medicine* 47, no. 18 (2008): 1573–1578, DOI: 10.2169/internalmedicine.47.0717, PMID: 18797115.

9. Maria Angeles Fuentes and others, "Lateral Functional Shift of the Mandible: Part II. Effects on Gene Expression in Condylar Cartilage," *American Journal of Orthodontics and Dentofacial Orthopedics* 123, no. 2 (2003): 160–166, DOI: 10.1067/mod.2003.6, PMID: 12594422.

Ch. 13: The Telltale Tongue

1. G. Dave Singh and James A. Krumholtz, *Epigenetic Orthodontics in Adults* (Chatsworth, CA: Smile Foundation, 2009), page 60; Melvin L. Moss, "The Functional Matrix Hypothesis Revisited: 2. The Role of an Osseous Connected Cellular Network," *American Journal of Orthodontics and Dentofacial Orthopedics* 112, no. 2 (1997): 221–226, DOI: *10.1016/S0889-5406(97)70249-X*, PMID: *9267235*.

2. Yu-Shu Huang and others, "Short Lingual Frenulum and Obstructive Sleep Apnea in Children," *International Journal of Pediatric Research* 1, no. 1 (2015), http://clinmedjournals.org/articles/ijpr/ijpr-1-003.pdf.

3. Academy of Orofacial Myofunctional Therapy, "Frequently Asked Questions and Answers in the Area of Orofacial Myofunctional Therapy" (Pacific Palisades, CA: Academy of Orofacial Myofunctional Therapy, 2014).

4. See note 2; Christian Guilleminault and others, "Pediatric OSA, Myo-facial Reeducation, and Facial Growth," *Journal of Sleep Research* 21, suppl. 1, (2012): 70.

5. Anna H. Messner and M. Lauren Lalakea, "Ankyloglossia: Controversies in Management," *International Journal of Pediatric Otorhinolaryngology* 54, no. 2–3 (2000): 123–131, DOI: *10.1016/S0165-5876(00)00359-1*, PMID: *10967382*.

6. Irene Queiroz Marchesan, "Lingual Frenum Protocol," *International Journal of Orofacial Myology* 38 (2012): 89–103, PMID: *23367525, http://cpal.edu.pe/info/2012 Marchesan Lingual Frenulum Protocol.pdf.*

7. Yu-Shu Huang and others, "Short Lingual Frenulum and Obstructive Sleep Apnea in Children," *International Journal of Pediatric Research* 1, no. 1 (2015), http://clinmedjournals.org/articles/ijpr/ijpr-1-003.pdf.

8. Macario Camacho and others, "Myofunctional Therapy to Treat Obstructive Sleep Apnea: A Systematic Review and Meta-analysis," *SLEEP* 38, no. 5 (2015): 669–675, DOI: 10.5665/sleep.4652, PMID: 25348130.

9. Academy of Orofacial Myofunctional Therapy, "Frequently Asked Questions and Answers in the Area of Orofacial Myofunctional Therapy", Pacific Palisades, CA, Academy of Orofacial Myofunctional Therapy (2014).

Ch. 14: Tongue-tie's Treachery

1. U.S. Department of Health and Human Services, Oral Health in America: A Report of the Surgeon General (Rockville, MD: U.S. Department of Health and Human Services, National Institute of Dental and Craniofacial

Research, National Institutes of Health, 2000), 10–11, Table 1.

2. Anahad O'Connor, "Sleep Apnea Tied to Increased Cancer Risk," *Well: Tara Parker-Pope on Health* (blog), *New York Times,* May 20, 2012, http://well.blogs.nytimes. com/2012/05/20/sleep-apnea-tied-to-increased-cancer-risk/.

3. F. Javier Nieto and others, "Sleep-Disordered Breathing and Cancer Mortality: Results from the Wisconsin Sleep Cohort Study," *American Journal of Respiratory and Critical Care Medicine* 186, no. 2 (2012): 190–194, DOI: 10.1164/rccm.201201-0130OC, PMID: 22610391.

Ch. 15: Achieving CPAP Freedom

1. Steven Y. Park, "How a Dentist Can Cure Your Sleep Apnea," *Dr. Park's Sleep Apnea Blog,* September 24, 2014, http://doctorstevenpark.com/tag/alf; also author of *Sleep Interrupted: A Physician Reveals the #1 Reason Why So Many of Us Are Sick and Tired* (New York: Jodev Press, LLC, 2009).

2. Xavier Barceló and others, "Oropharyngeal Examination to Predict Sleep Apnea Severity," *Archives of Otolaryngology — Head & Neck Surgery* 137, no. 10 (2011): 990–996, DOI: 10.1001/archoto.2011.176, PMID: 22006776.

3. G. Dave Singh, "Guest Editorial on the Etiology and Significance of Palatal and Mandibular Tori," *CRANIO: The Journal of Craniomandibular & Sleep Practice* 28, no. 4 (2010): 213–215, DOI: 10.1179/crn.2010.030, PMID: 21032973.

4. SM Banabilh, AH Suzina, S Dinsuhaimi, AR Samsudin, GD Singh."Dental Arch Morphology in South-East

Asian Adults with Obstructive Sleep Apnoea: Geometric Morphometrics," *Journal of Oral Rehabilitation* 36, no. 3 (2009): 184–192, DOI: 10.1111/j.1365-2842.2008.01915.x, PMID: 19207445.

5. Murray Johns, "What the Epworth Sleepiness Scale Is and How to Use It," The Epworth Sleepiness Scale, http:// epworthsleepinessscale.com/about-epworth-sleepiness/.

6. G. Dave Singh, S. Wendling, and R. Chandrashekhar, "Midfacial Development in Adult Obstructive Sleep Apnea," *Dentistry Today,* June 30, 2011, 124–127, http://www.dentistrytoday.com/dental-medicine/dental-sleep-medicine/5674-midfacial-development-in-adult-obstructive-sleep-apnea.

Ch. 16: Stem Cell Activation

1. U.S. Department of Health and Human Services, *Oral Health in America: A Report of the Surgeon General* (Rockville, MD: U.S. Department of Health and Human Services, National Institute of Dental and Craniofacial Research, National Institutes of Health, 2000), http://www. nidcr.nih.gov/DataStatistics/SurgeonGeneral/sgr/welcome. htm.

2. Vincent G. Kokich, "The Biology of Sutures," chap. 4 in Craniosynostosis: Diagnosis, Evaluation, and Management, ed. M. Michael Cohen Jr. (New York: Raven Press, 1986), 81–103.

3. Lynne A. Opperman, "Cranial Sutures as Intramembranous Bone Growth Sites," *Developmental Dynamics* 219, no. 4 (2000): 472–485, DOI:

10.1002/1097-0177(2000)9999:9999<::AID-DVDY1073>3.0.CO;2-F, PMID: 11084647.

4. V. Kokich, "The Biology of Sutures," chap. 4 in Craniosynostosis: Diagnosis, Evaluation, and Management, ed. M. Michael Cohen Jr. (New York: Raven Press, 1986), 94.

5. Cinderella de Pollack and others, "Increased Bone Formation and Osteoblastic Cell Phenotype in Premature Cranial Suture Ossification (Craniosynostosis)," *Journal of Bone and Mineral Research* 11, no. 3 (1996): 401–407, DOI: 10.1002/jbmr.5650110314, PMID: 8852951.

6. G. Dave Singh and James A. Krumholtz, *Epigenetic Orthodontics in Adults* (Chatsworth, CA: Smile Foundation, 2009), 45.

7. G. Dave Singh and James A. Krumholtz, *Epigenetic Orthodontics in Adults* (Chatsworth, CA: Smile Foundation, 2009), 45.

8. C.A. McCulloch, "Origins and Functions of Cells Essential for Periodontal Repair: The Role of Fibroblasts in Tissue Homeostasis," *Oral Diseases* 1, no. 4 (1995): 271–278, DOI: 10.1111/j.1601-0825.1995.tb00193.x, PMID: 8705836.

9. Wen-Lang Lin, Christopher A.G. McCulloch, and Moon-Il Cho, "Differentiation of Periodontal Ligament Fibroblasts into Osteoblasts During Socket Healing After Tooth Extraction in the Rat," *The Anatomical Record* 240, no. 4 (1994): 492–506, DOI: 10.1002/ar.1092400407, PMID: 7879901.

10. Byoung-Moo Seo and others, "Investigation of Multipotent Postnatal Stem Cells from Human Periodontal Ligament,"

Lancet 364, no. 9429 (2004): 149–155, DOI: 10.1016/
S0140-6736(04)16627-0, PMID: 15246727.

11. Jun Isaka and others, "Participation of Periodontal
Ligament Cells with Regeneration of Alveolar Bone,"
Journal of Periodontology 72, no. 3 (2001): 314–323, DOI:
10.1902/jop.2001.72.3.314, PMID: 11327058.

12. G. Dave Singh and James A. Krumholtz, *Epigenetic
Orthodontics in Adults* (Chatsworth, CA: Smile
Foundation, 2009), 278. G.

13. Dave Singh, T.M. Griffin, and R. Chandrashekhar,
"Biomimetic Oral Appliance Therapy in Adults with
Mild to Moderate Obstructive Sleep Apnea," Austin
Journal of Sleep Disorders 1, no. 1 (2014): 5, http://
austinpublishinggroup.com/sleep-disorders/fulltext/ajsd-v1-
id1002.php.

14. G. Dave Singh; Tara Griffin; Samuel E Cress Biomimetic
Oral Appliance Therapy in Adults with Severe Obstructive
Sleep Apnea Sleep Disorder & Therapy Volume 5 Issue 1
(2016)

15. Liao F, Singh GD. Effects of Biomimetic Oral Appliance
Therapy on Epworth Scores in Adults with Obstructive
Sleep ApneaJ Dent Sleep Med. 3(3), 98, 2016. http://dx.doi.
org/10.15331/jdsm.5996

16. Murray Johns, "What the Epworth Sleepiness Scale Is
and How to Use It," The Epworth Sleepiness Scale, http://
epworthsleepinessscale.com/about-epworth-sleepiness/.

Ch. 17: Promoting Children's Holistic Mouth Development and Full Genetic Expression

1. Yu-Shu Huang and Christian Guilleminault, "Pediatric Obstructive Sleep Apnea and the Critical Role of Oral-Facial Growth: Evidences," *Frontiers in Neurology* 3 (2012): 184, DOI: 10.3389/fneur.2012.00184, PMID: 23346072.

2. See note 1.

3. "What Is the Difference Between Epigenetics and Epigenomics?" Epigenesys, http://www.epigenesys.eu/it/public/faq-common/111-what-is-the-difference-between-epigenetics-and-epigenomics.

4. "Epigenomics," National Human Genome Research Institute, http://www.genome.gov/27532724.

5. Christian Guilleminault and others, "Sleep Apnea in Eight Children," *Pediatrics* 58, no. 1 (1976): 23–30, http://pediatrics.aappublications.org/content/58/1/23, PMID: 934781.)

6. Rakesh Bhattacharjee and others, "Adenotonsillectomy Outcomes in Treatment of Obstructive Sleep Apnea in Children: A Multicenter Retrospective Study," *American Journal of Respiratory and Critical Care Medicine* 182, no. 5 (2010): 676–683, DOI: 10.1164/rccm.200912-1930OC, PMID: 20448096.

7. See note 1.

8. Viola M. Frymann, D.O., Relation of disturbances of craniosacral mechanism to symptomatology of the newborn: Study of 1,250 infants. *J.A.O.A.* 65 (1966), 1059-1075.

9. Christian Guilleminault, Yu-shu Huang, Stacey Quo, Pierre-Jean Monteyrol, Cheng-hui Lin, Teenage sleep-disordered breathing: Recurrence of syndrome, Sleep Medicine 14 (2013) 37–44.

10. Aelred C. Fonder, "Dental Distress Syndrome Quantified," *Basal Facts* 9, no. 4 (1987): 141–167, http://www. betterhealththruresearch.com/OldSite/DDS.pdf.

11. Enlow D, Moyers R, Merow W, Handbook of Facial Development, W. Saunders, 1976

12. John Flutter, The Etiology of Malocclusion: http://www. fogvedo.hu/downloads/tudomany_cikk/The_Aetiology_of_ Malocclusion%5B1%5D.pdf.

13. Bresolin D, Shapiro PA, Shapiro GG, Chapko MK, Dassel S. Mouth Breathing in Allergic Children: Its Relationship to Dentofacial Development. *American Journal of Orthodontics* 1983.

14. Egil P. Harvold, DDS Ph.D.,L.L.D.Brittta S. Tamer, DDS, Kevin Varervik, DDS., and George Chierici, DDS - American Journal of Orthodontics Vol 79. No. 4 April, 1981.

15. Rappai M1, Collop N, Kemp S, deShazo R. The nose and sleep-disordered breathing: what we know and what we do not know. Chest. 2003 Dec;124(6):2309-23.

16. Chang MC, Enlow DH , Papsidero M , Broadbent BH Jr , Oyen O , Sabat M, Developmental Effects of Impaired Breathing in the Face of the Growing Child, The Angle Orthodontist, October, 1988, 58(4),309-320.

17. Gill Rapley and Tracey Murkett , Baby-Led Weaning: http://www.amazon.com/Baby-Led-Weaning-Essential-Introducing-Confident/dp/161519021X

18. Dr. Lawrence Wilson, Food Sensitivities or Intolerance.

19. Patrick McKeown, Close Your Mouth: Stop Asthma, Hay Fever, and Nasal Congestion Permanently. Buteyko Books, Galway 2004.

20. Environmental Work Group, Cord Blood Study, July, 2005.

21. Jonathan M.P. Howat, Chiropractic Cranio Fascial Dynamics, Chapter 2. Cranial Communication Systems, Oxford UK 2009.

22. See Note 8.

23. Francis M. Pottenger Jr., *Pottenger's Cats: A Study in Nutrition,* 2nd ed. (Lemon Grove, CA: Price-Pottenger Nutrition Foundation, 1995.

Ch. 19: Holistic Mouth Checkup

1. David G. Simons, Janet G. Travell, and Lois S. Simons, "Perpetuating Factors," chap. 4 in Myofascial Pain and Dysfunction: The Trigger Point Manual, vol. 1, Upper Half of Body, 2nd ed. (Baltimore, MD: Lippincott Williams & Wilkins, 1998).

2. Vishesh K. Kanpur and Edward M. Weaver, "Filling in the Pieces of the Sleep Apnea-Hypertension Puzzle," *Journal of the American Medical Association* 307, no. 20 (2012): 2197–2198, DOI: 10.1001/jama.2012.5039, PMID: 22618928.

3. Mary L. Adams, MS, MPH, Angela J. Deokar, MPH, Lynda
    A. Anderson, PhD, Valerie J. Edwards, PhD, Self-Reported
    Increased Confusion or Memory Loss and Associated
    Functional Difficulties Among Adults Aged ≥60 Years —
    21 States, 2011. Morbidity and Mortality Weekly Report,
    May 10, 2013 / 62(18);347-350, Div of Population Health,
    National Center for Chronic Disease Prevention and Health
    Promotion, CDC.

4. Angela R. Kamer and others, "Periodontal Inflammation in
    Relation to Cognitive Function in an Older Danish Adult
    Population," *Journal of Alzheimer's Disease* 28, no. 3
    (2012): 613–624, DOI: 10.3233/JAD-2011-102004, PMID:
    22045483.

5. Jana R. Cooke and others, "Sustained Use of CPAP Slows
    Deterioration of Cognition, Sleep, and Mood in Patients
    with Alzheimer's Disease and Obstructive Sleep Apnea:
    A Preliminary Study," *Journal of Clinical Sleep Medicine*
    5, no. 4 (2009): 305–309, http://www.aasmnet.org/jcsm/
    ViewAbstract.aspx?pid=27538, PMID: 19968005.

6. Ide M, Harris M, Stevens A, Sussams R, Hopkins V,
    Culliford D, et al. (2016) Periodontitis and Cognitive
    Decline in Alzheimer's Disease. PLoS ONE 11(3):
    e0151081. doi:10.1371/journal.pone.0151081

7. Dementia is the Most Costly Disease in America,
    Alzheimer's Association: http://act.alz.org/site/
    MessageViewer?dlv_id=101541&em_id=80007.0

Ch. 20: From Teeth To Mouth: The Next Paradigm Shift

1. What Is A Paradigm Shift: http://www.taketheleap.com/
    define.html

2. Jo-Dee L. Lattimore, David S. Celermajer, and Ian Wilcox, "Obstructive Sleep Apnea and Cardiovascular Disease," *Journal of the American College of Cardiology* 41, no. 9 (2003): 1429–1437, DOI: 10.1016/S0735-1097(03)00184-0, PMID: 12742277.

3. U.S. Centers for Disease Control and Prevention FastStats: http://www.cdc.gov/nchs/fastats/leading-causes-of-death.htm

4. Dementia is the Most Costly Disease in America, Alzheimer's Association: http://act.alz.org/site/MessageViewer?dlv_id=101541&em_id=80007.0

5. Michael D. Hurd, Ph.D., Paco Martorell, Ph.D., Adeline Delavande, Ph.D., Kathleen J. Mullen, Ph.D., and Kenneth M. Langa, M.D., Ph.D., Monetary Costs of Dementia in the United States. N Engl J Med 2013; 368:1326-1334April 4, 2013DOI: 10.1056/NEJMsa1204629

6. U.S. Department of Health and Human Services. *Oral Health in America: A Report of the Surgeon General.* Rockville, MD: U.S. Department of Health and Human Services, National Institute of Dental and Craniofacial Research, National Institutes of Health, 2000. Executive Summary, part IV.

7. Delta Dental Oral Health and Well-Being Survey of 2014. "Survey Finds Shortcomings in Americans'Dental Health Habits," Delta Dental, Sept. 23, 2014, https://www.deltadental.com/Public/NewsMedia/NewsReleaseDentalSurveyFindsShortcomings_201409.jsp.)

8. See Note 3.

9. See Note 3.

10. *National Call to Action to Promote Oral Health,* Richard Carmona, MD. U.S. Department of Health and Human Services. Rockville, MD. U.S. Department of Health and Human Services, Public Health Service, National Institutes of Health, National Institute of Dental and Craniofacial Research. NIH Publication No. 03-5303, http://www.nidcr.nih.gov/DataStatistics/SurgeonGeneral/ NationalCalltoAction/nationalcalltoaction.htm

11. "Diabetes? Heart Disease? Osteoporosis? Your Dentist May Know Before You Do," Delta Dental, September 2014, https://www.deltadentalins.com/oral_health/dentists-detect. html.No. 03-5303, Spring 2003.

Made in the USA
Las Vegas, NV
28 December 2022